WHEN WOMEN SEXUALLY ABUSE MEN

WHEN WOMEN SEXUALLY ABUSE MEN

The Hidden Side of Rape, Stalking, Harassment, and Sexual Assault

PHILIP W. COOK
WITH TAMMY L. HODO, PHD

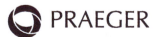 PRAEGER

AN IMPRINT OF ABC-CLIO, LLC
Santa Barbara, California • Denver, Colorado • Oxford, England

Library of Congress Cataloging-in-Publication Data

Cook, Philip W., 1948–
  When women sexually abuse men : the hidden side of rape, stalking, harassment, and sexual assault / Philip W. Cook with Tammy L. Hodo, PhD.
    pages cm
  Includes bibliographical references and index.
  ISBN 978-0-313-39729-5 (hardcopy : alk. paper) — ISBN 978-0-313-39730-1 (ebook) 1. Male sexual abuse victims—United States. 2. Abused men—United States. 3. Abused husbands—United States. 4. Abusive women—United States. 5. Family violence—United States. I. Hodo, Tammy L. II. Title.
  HV6561.C663 2013
  364.15'3208110973—dc23   2013010516

ISBN: 978-0-313-39729-5
EISBN: 978-0-313-39730-1

17 16 15 14   3 4 5

This book is also available on the World Wide Web as an eBook.
Visit www.abc-clio.com for details.

Praeger
An Imprint of ABC-CLIO, LLC

ABC-CLIO, LLC
130 Cremona Drive, P.O. Box 1911
Santa Barbara, California 93116-1911

This book is printed on acid-free paper ∞

Manufactured in the United States of America

Copyright Acknowledgments

The authors and publisher gratefully acknowledge permission for use of the following material:

Colleen O'Brien. "NW Woman Editor Charged with Identity Theft, Cyberstalking." KXLY TV Spokane, Washington, July 12, 2011. Copyright © 2011, KXLY TV.

Martin Fiebert, PhD. "References Examining Men as Victims of Women's Sexual Coercion." Annotated bibliography. Permission granted by author. http://. cottal.org/LBDUK/referecnes_examining_men_as_vic.htm.

Tara Palmatier, PhD. "Female Stalkers—What Is Stalking and Can Men Be Stalked by Women?" Permission granted by author. http://www.shrink4men. com/ February 8, 2011.

B.H. Hoff (2011). "National Study: More Men than Women Victims of Intimate Partner Physical Violence, Psychological Aggression. Over 40% of victims of severe physical violence are men." *Men Web*, online journal. Permission granted by author. http://www.batteredmen.com/NISVS.htm.

Malcolm George, MD. "From Rape to Something More Difficult to Contemplate." Article prepared for this volume, March 6, 1998. Used by permission.

Rosemary Purcell, BA, M Psych., Michele Pathé, MBBS, FRANZCP, and Paul E. Mullen, MBBS, DSc, FRC. "A Study of Women Who Stalk," *American Journal of Psychiatry* 158:2056–2060, December 2001, American Psychiatric Association. Reprinted with permission.

J. Reid Meloy, PhD, and Cynthia Boyd, PhD. "Female Stalkers and Their Victims." *Journal of the American Academy of Psychiatry Law* 31: 211–19, 2003.

Analysis of NISVS research and Correspondence with Centers for Disease Control and Prevention and Analysis of Department of Education Sexual Assault on Campus Directive. Stop Abusive and Violent Environments (SAVE). www.saveservices.org. Reprinted with permission.

Contents

Acknowledgments

A ny book is a collaborative effort—a fact that is paid tribute to by most authors. This book is no exception to that rule. This tribute must start with a simple note by my first (and only) literary agent, John Harney of Boston, who, a number of years ago, helped with the first edit for the first edition of *Abused Men: The Hidden Side of Domestic Violence*. He said, "Cut these paragraphs—it is a different subject that belongs in another book." My editor for that volume, Nancy Wolf, also encouraged a book on this subject, and I am also very grateful that she gave me some essential keys to better writing. Malcolm George, MD, of London, in interviews conducted for that book, was very enthusiastic that another book was needed, and as referenced in this volume, essential to this work. Dr. George passed away in 2013 and this book is dedicated to his memory. Martin Fiebert, PhD, of Long Beach, California is also acknowledged in the text, and his work is especially critical. There are many other researchers, therapists, sociologists, and journalists whose work we have drawn from, and we strived very hard to acknowledge all in the notes or in the text and quote or paraphrased them accurately. As noted, a special thank you again to those who gave us permission to quote extensively from their work. Thank you for deciding to tackle difficult issues in your research and reporting. Warren Farrell, PhD, of California, author of many volumes, including the essential *Myth of Male Power* has been supportive of my work and it should be known that he was the first to publish a book regarding many of the issues and subjects raised in this volume. I wish I had his gift for the pithy and appropriate 'ah-hah' phrase. The organization Stop Abusive and Violent Environments is recognized for helpfully agreeing to provide correspondence, reports, and analysis.

Thank you! Harry Crouch, Stanley Green, Ron Henry, Howard Fradkin, and others too numerous to name, are to be thanked for their continued work in raising awareness about these issues. R. L. McNeely, PhD, JD of Milwaukee, Wisconsin, has been a longtime personal friend, always supportive and most key for this effort in referring me to the collaborator for this volume, Tammy Hodo, PhD. Last, but by no means the least, this book is dedicated to my wife, Nadine Smith-Cook. The gift of real encouragement and belief is wonderful and rare.

—Philip W. Cook

I would like to thank Philip Cook for asking me to assist him with this very important topic and project. I definitely have learned how difficult and time-consuming putting a book together can be, but know that this topic is a relatively new phenomenon in academic research and is an important issue that needs to be brought to the forefront. I would also like to thank R. L. McNeely, PhD, JD and Ms. Pauli Taylor-Boyd of the University of Wisconsin-Milwaukee for introducing me to Mr. Cook and tossing my name in the hat for an opportunity to work on this important topic. To my husband, Linnen, and son, Jonah, I want to thank you for your patience and understanding while I was working on this project.

—Tammy L. Hodo

Introduction

All truth passes through three stages. First, it is ridiculed. Second,
it is violently opposed. Third, it is accepted as being self-evident.
                                                    —Arthur Schopenhauer

The dictum of 19th-century philosopher Schopenhauer is relevant
to this volume due to the reception of my previous work, *Abused
Men: The Hidden Side of Domestic Violence*, first published in 1997
and in an updated second edition in 2009. As discussed in that book,
the change in general attitudes among the news media and the general
public cannot be precisely charted, but it can be chronicled. It certainly
follows the path that Schopenhauer outlined. This includes the fact that,
at first, there was indeed heavy ridicule of even the idea that such men
exist and have similar outcomes to women in the same situation. There
was, indeed, violent opposition toward early researchers such as Richard Gelles, Murray Straus, and Suzanne Steinmetz, but also toward the
founder of the battered woman's movement, Erin Pizzey. For me, such
violent opposition was rare, though suppression of the presentation of
even academic research, let alone discussion in domestic violence conferences or by advocacy groups, remains a fairly common phenomenon.
The evidence for that is legion even today and tends to follow the path
of the Yiddish proverb: "Half the truth is a good as a whole lie." That
is, evidence for the existence of abused men is now mentioned as a fact
whereas before it was most often neglected entirely, but it is still most
often and quite deliberately downplayed by intentionally comparing different types of research results to achieve the desired result. Certainly,
while services for such men are increasing, they are still rare. However,
while it is not always self-evident that such men exist and need at least

some attention to their plight, it is certainly much more widely accepted than in 1997. These issues are explored more fully in the second edition of *Abused Men*.

It is to be expected therefore that this volume, exploring—as *Abused Men* did—a heretofore mainly unexamined aspect of human behavior, will elicit controversy. This is a book intended for a general readership rather than a strictly academic one, though it may prove useful in that regard as well. It is intended to provide the first-ever comprehensive overview of research, news accounts, and personal stories, of a particular kind of adult female criminal and aberrant behavior and its effects on adult men. It is not intended to always *equate* the rape of a man by a woman, for example, with the rape of a woman by a man. There are differences, both in the effect and consequences of such an act as rape or other crimes and behaviors, as well as similarities. These differences and similarities will be explored in this volume.

Cases of adult women and teachers sexually abusing boys have become a fairly frequent item in the news. News cycles wax and wane, but certainly, it can be said that there has been an increase in this kind of news story in the last 10 years. There are books as well as helping and nonprofit organizations dealing with the trauma of childhood sexual abuse by women and men. The reader is advised that this book does not deal with such childhood traumas. This volume deals with the shocking and true accounts of *adult* women stalking, sexually assaulting, sexually harassing, and even raping *adult* men. How men can be raped by adult women with or without a sexual arousal by the male victim is explained. An estimation of the extent of male rape by adult women is provided. This book does not just deal with rape, however, but a whole range of crimes and behaviors including sexual assaults, aggressive and unwanted sexual advances, sexual harassment, and stalking by women against men. This is the first book to look at all of these issues in one place. Astonishing information is revealed, including the finding that a majority of studies have found that *equal* numbers of men and women felt that they have been threatened or pressured into having sex when they did not want to. You will also learn that stalking and sexual harassment by women against men is on the rise, and now exceeds the reverse in one category of stalking. You will hear personal accounts from males and learn what is and is not being done to deal with a little known type of crime and behavior that is definitely on the increase. The issue of false accusations of rape and other sexual crimes is not neglected. Evidence is provided to illustrate that such falsehoods are simply another type of sexual assault. The reader will follow true crime stories that reveal, at times, horrifying acts, and new information is provided as to how often these crimes and types of sexually coercive behavior actually occur. This volume reveals how the victims, their friends, and family deal with these events while also providing useful help for victims. We will also examine how society and the media respond or fail to respond to these events. Significant public policy issues are examined in a number of areas.

The author is assisted in this volume by respected criminologist Tammy Hodo, PhD. *When Women Sexually Abuse Men: The Hidden Side of Rape, Stalking, Harassment, and Sexual Assault* may eventually change how society views and attempts to deal with these types of human behaviors.

CHAPTER 1

When Women Rape Men

Rape and Torture in Spokane

Prosecuting attorney Jon Love had a problem, and it was not a lack of evidence. In fact, in his years as a prosecutor and on the other side, as a criminal defense attorney, he had never had a rape case in which there was more evidence than this one. There was "a ton" of forensic evidence from the crime scene and on the victim's body; there was an eyewitness who turned on the accomplice, and, a very rare thing in a rape case—there were neighbors who had actually seen abusive behavior by the defendant prior to the actual rape. The defendant was unrepentant and unsympathetic. And there were horrifying pictures of the victim's injuries that would turn the heart of even the coldest juror.

Jon Love should have been the most confident of prosecutors, but he was not.

The reason Love was worried the jury would not convict was because the rape victim was a man and the rapist was a woman. As many as five of the original panel of jurors in his medium-sized city, "women who were part of the beehive hairdo set"—as he called them—had said in jury seating questioning that they did not believe a rape could be possible or proved.

It was almost enough to make him wish there had not been a rookie cop on duty the night the victim was discovered nearly a year earlier. A hardened veteran officer would have likely told the man to go sleep it off somewhere. But, the rookie bent down to actually listen when the man mumbled something about not being able to move fast because of the burns.

The mumbling man was Ron Varga. He was 41 years old, childless, a highway toll booth collector in New Jersey. He had been living for six years with his 36-year-old common-law wife, Diane Eunice Ickhoff. Ron and Diane had become close friends with Theresa Spickler-Bowe, a woman about their age. Diane and Theresa became particularly close, so when Theresa decided to move to Spokane, Washington, Diane told Ron she was leaving him to go with Theresa. Diane hoped for a more interesting life and thought Theresa and her husband, Bill Bowe, could find her a job. Ron was upset. His toll job was OK and steady work, and he thought they were building a life together. However, the prospect of making a new life someplace quite different was not unappealing, and maybe there would be a better life out West. He could not convince Diane to stay, so he decided to move to Spokane with her.

Theresa was not keen on Ron moving with them at first, but decided that it would be okay for both of them to share an apartment with her and her husband for a while. Plans were made and Theresa left for Spokane to join her husband Bill, who was already living there. Ron and Diane followed a short time later by bus.

From the very beginning, things did not work out as planned. Ron and Diane arrived in Spokane in August. They had lost their entire luggage on the bus trip and arrived with just the clothes on their back and very little money. Later that year, Spokane experienced one of the harshest winters on record, and a major ice storm even got Spokane declared a federal disaster area. It was colder than New Jersey, and a lot windier.

Bill Bowe had a ground-level, two-bedroom, one-bath apartment in a low-rent part of town. Instead of sharing a bedroom with her husband, Theresa was sleeping on the living room couch. Bill was gone a lot, sometimes absent for days at a time. He worked at a hotel during the day and as a janitor at night, and he would often sleep at the hotel between his two jobs instead of coming back to the apartment. Theresa wanted the other bedroom kept free for storage, laundry, and other uses. Bill had "her" bedroom and his comings and goings disturbed her. She also said her "bad back," which prevented her from working, made the couch more comfortable than the bed. At first, Ron and Diane slept in the second bedroom, but after a month or so, they were told they had to sleep on the living room floor.

Theresa told them that she would not tolerate them "mooching" on her, and that Ron or Diane had to go to work immediately to pay their share of the rent and expenses. Theresa told Diane that she had to make Ron obey her and "act right," and that she would help her see that this happened.

The threesome got to know their neighbors, who thought that Theresa was nice and she certainly kept a clean and tidy house. There were pleasant pictures and interesting curios. They described Diane as nice, but a little odd, and Ron was thought to be a simple quiet guy who was reserved, shy, and submissive to Diane and Theresa. Some wondered if he was not somehow mentally retarded. Later, some became convinced he was. It helped them rationalize some of the things they saw, and felt it would help explain some of the "control" measures taken by Theresa and Diane.

Ron went to work for a temporary agency that handled mostly manual labor. The work was tough, especially as he is slight of build (only 130 pounds and five feet, eight inches). Diane is a very petite woman, 115 pounds, while Theresa, though not much taller than Diane's five feet, five inches, was big boned and large, at about 250 pounds. Ron worked at the labor jobs nearly every day. He showed up early to get on the job board, and his supervisors thought he was a hard worker. He eventually got a second job at a fast-food hamburger chain. Diane started working as well, eventually holding two jobs, one in a grocery store and another helping out in a deli.

Theresa had to "approve" of their jobs before they could take them, to make sure, she said, that they were pulling in their share of the expenses. The rent was just $450 a month—by Spokane standards of the time, not exceptionally low, but at the lower end of the scale.

Eventually, Theresa got a further reduction in the rent by having Ron shovel snow around the complex and having him do some landscape work and small repairs for the landlord. She handled all the bills for the household and constantly complained that Ron and Diane were taking advantage of her. Theresa and Diane gave notes to Ron on a daily basis. They told him when he was to report to work, when he was to come home, when and where to deposit his checks, where to go to buy groceries, and what errands to take care of. When the police eventually found him, they found one of these notes in his pocket.

Theresa began a campaign of disparaging anything that Ron did, and she began to train Diane in how to "take care of him." The neighbors came over less and less, until they stopped coming over altogether. They sensed coolness from Theresa and Diane, and they began to hear loud yelling and arguments from the apartment. Toward the end of the year, one neighbor got into the habit of wearing earplugs to bed—there were awful sounds coming from next door.

Theresa said she was dissatisfied with the sleeping arrangements and that she did not want Ron and Diane to share the living room any more. It was too crowded, and they got in her way when she wanted to get up from the couch. Ron was to sleep on the uncarpeted kitchen floor.

At first, he had a sleeping bag, but after a month, he was allowed only blankets. By about the end of the year, he was sleeping only in his underwear or naked, directly on the bare floor.

His food intake began to be controlled. If he burped during dinnertime, his food was taken away. Eventually, for passing gas or burping, not only was his food taken away, but either Theresa, Diane, or both of them would hit him. He was sometimes force-fed by Diane or Theresa and given only small, child-sized portions. Sometimes his food would be thrown on the floor and he had to eat it with his hands or lap at it, like a dog. At his fast-food job, he had access to food, but if he was discovered by Theresa or Diane to have eaten there, he would be in trouble at home. When he came home from work, Diane would chain him to her waist. He was not to move unless directed by Theresa or Diane. Any small transgression was a reason for a beating; sometimes, both women jumped on his legs.

The neighbors described seeing him being forced to shovel the snow with a dog chain around his neck and very little clothing on. He was allowed only cold showers. His bathroom privileges were restricted. He was made to wear only a homemade diaper.

If he could not hold his urine or bowel movement and soiled his diaper, the women began to burn him for this violation of the "rules." At first, a butter knife was heated up with hot water and applied to his chest. Later, they heated it up on the stove burner and applied it all over his body, including his buttocks. They also heated up a large flat metal spatula and burned him with that. Ron still carries the burn scars, and the peculiar marks made by the spatula blade can clearly be seen even today.

If he did not do a good job shoveling snow or the two women became displeased by something, he was made to stand out in the patio in the snow, dressed only in his diapers. He had to carry out the garbage in his bare feet. The neighbors noticed the tracks in the snow. Despite this evidence that the neighbors noticed, and the yelling and occasional sounds of agony from the apartment, no one ever called the police.

Two of his fast-food coworkers testified about the changes they noted in Ron from the time he started working until a few days before he was discovered by police. At the end, he was withdrawn, emaciated, and would not make eye contact. The neighbors agreed with this characterization.

Ron was made to hold a rake handle over his head for long periods of time as punishment. On at least one occasion, when he could no longer hold it up, Diane and Theresa took it from him and made him bend over, and then rammed the rake handle violently up his anus causing internal lacerations.

After one of the rapes with the rake handle (investigators were never sure just how many times it happened) around the first of January, Ron Varga was forced by Diane and Theresa to drink a large quantity of alcohol. He could not go to work that day. He was bleeding from blows around his head. By now, he weighed just 116 pounds. Prosecuting attorney Patti Connolly-Walker described him as looking like someone from a concentration camp. In a sense, he was—the gulag of Diane and Theresa. After being force-fed the alcohol, the women ejected him from the apartment. It was late at night and having nowhere to go, he walked a few miles to an alcohol treatment center called First Steps. He fell asleep on a couch. Because First Steps is a drop-in-only center with no sleeping accommodations, visitors are not permitted to sleep there. The staff tried to get him up, but could not rouse him. They called police to remove yet another typical drunk who was violating the no-sleepover rule.

Perhaps for the first time in his life, Ron Varga was lucky that night. A rookie cop happened to be one of the responding officers. The veteran officer paired with the rookie told prosecutors that he probably would not have taken the time that the rookie did. He noticed a bit of dried blood in Varga's hair and around his face and neck, but he had seen that kind of thing before in a falling-down drunk and would have just put him back on the street if he could walk, taken him home, or taken him to detox at the jail. The rookie, though, began to ask Ron questions; he thought he might be injured. Ron was unable to get up off the couch without assistance. He mumbled something about the burns as reason he could not move quickly. When the officer asked him, "What burns?" Ron tried to pull his shirt out at the neck so the officer could see. The shirt had stuck to his burns and pieces of flesh were being pulled off. The rookie noticed further wounds on his ears and neck, as well as bruises on his arms. The two officers then called for assistance and a corporal arrived to take photographs of the injuries. When they got his shirt off, all three described the injuries as among the worst they had ever seen. The two responding officers took him to the emergency room. Ron had a broken nose, broken ribs, and frostbite, was covered with burns and bruises, and had sustained severe damage to his rectal area.

At the eventual trial of Theresa Spickler-Bowe, the doctor who examined Ron in the emergency room was asked by prosecutor Patti Connolly-Walker to diagram, on a body chart, the areas of injury. The head of emergency medicine told the court, "It would be easier to diagram the areas *not* injured."

Police moved quickly to question the neighbors, as well as Bill Bowe, Theresa, and Diane. Bowe claimed he knew nothing of what was going on since he was rarely at the apartment. He was eventually cleared and not charged with any crime. Diane quickly agreed to cooperate with prosecutors to make a case against Theresa. Prosecutors told her they would recommend to the judge an "exceptional" sentence of 12 years for first-degree rape and second-degree assault for cooperating, but if Diane did not plead guilty and cooperate in the case against Theresa, and she was convicted at trial, she could receive a sentence of 20 years. Diane's sentence hearing was held after Theresa's trial. Judge Gregory Sypolt, however, did not buy Diane's tearful story that Theresa made her torture and rape Ron. He ignored the prosecutors' recommendation for 12 years for both crimes. She was given 10 years and 5 months in prison for first-degree rape and an additional 10 years for second-degree assault.

Diane's sentencing was in the future, however, and meanwhile, they had her cooperation against Theresa. Theresa Spickler-Bowe vehemently claimed that Diane did everything and that Theresa herself was not much involved. She was free on bail for a time after her arrest, but then, she was arrested for attempting to flee on bond when she tried to sell a car and made some statements about getting out of town. Prosecutors Jon Love and Patti Connolly-Walker began to question potential jurors in June. Love was not worried about the forensic evidence. They had the rake handle with traces of feces and a human hair still on it. They had the horrifying pictures of Ron Varga's condition and the medical records and doctors' testimony. They had the chain used to tie him up. Besides the forensic evidence, they also had the neighbors and coworkers testimony, and they had Diane ready to spill everything she knew.

Love and Walker's biggest problem was with the victim and their concern about sexism on the jury. Ron Varga could not remember much. He did not recall details and had apparently blocked nearly everything out. He was not very clear on who had done what and when, except that both women had done things to him. Still, this was understandable with someone who had been tortured as he had been, and they felt they could make the jury see that his memory lapse was not unusual. They eventually felt fairly comfortable with the jury they got, which included two nurses and a volunteer for a sexual abuse prevention network. In the back of Love's mind, however, was the concern about the "beehive hairdo ladies" and their belief that a man could never be raped.

The women felt that a man could always escape a situation, whereas a woman would not be able to, because of economic circumstances and submissive behavior. Men just are not that way . . . it does not happen . . . could not happen . . . , according to their statements in jury questioning.

At trial, though, Love got a big gift from the defense. Theresa testified. She was unbelievable and unsympathetic and clearly of a domineering A-type, as Love hoped he could get her to reveal. The tears flowed, but it did her no good.

The evidence was overwhelming and the vote was unanimous for conviction on both counts. Theresa Spickler-Bowe was sentenced in 1997 to 10 years on both counts of first-degree rape and second-degree assault. Because Judge Sypolt refused to accept the plea bargain, Diane and Theresa ended up with the same sentence—20 years in prison.

Ron Varga returned to New Jersey and his job on the New Jersey turnpike. Patti Connolly-Walker is still a prosecuting attorney in Spokane County and also works as an attorney for the City of Spokane. Jon Love went to work for the Immigration and Naturalization Service in San Antonio, Texas.

After the verdict, there were a few calls from the national news media and television productions, but as far as Love can determine, nothing came of them. The news media in Spokane gave heavy coverage to the case, and the news media in Seattle covered some developments, such as the arrest and the verdict, but it was mainly ignored by the news media elsewhere—even in the neighboring state of Oregon.[1]

In one sense, this particular case fits the narrow parameters of how male rape by an adult woman could occur as an extremely rare incident, with the use of an object or objects.

Not So Rare?

Former prosecutor Love, however, has an entirely different view. He does not think it is that rare at all.

There have been many cases that I am aware of in [in Seattle where he formerly worked] in which the police suspected and told me that there was something more going on. That while they were investigating a domestic violence case in which the woman had been the primary assaulter they suspected that the man had been sexually abused as well. They would find evidence, feces on a dildo or other object and question the man about it, but he would never admit it. He would hang his head, and just not talk about it. It was difficult enough to get them to admit that they were being physically attacked by a woman, but to get them to say that they were sexually abused as well . . . that's just too emasculating . . . they can't do it.

Love recalls the case of a biker couple. "I was the public defender for her. I am sorry to say that I did my job and got her off, because the jury believed that he had consented once to rough sex and so when he objected to another time it didn't matter. That was rape, but she wasn't charged with rape, but assault. It happens. Men can be raped, have been raped, we just don't hear about it."[2]

The late (2011) Patricia Overberg was the former executive director of the Valley Oasis Shelter in Lancaster, California. For many years, it was the only shelter in the United States that accepted male victims of domestic violence. She has little doubt that in intimate partner relationships, men can be, and have been, raped by adult women. Stranger rapes are less common she believes, but it does happen.

I know of one case for example, a man was hitchhiking in California and he was picked up by two women in a van. They pulled over, held him down, and though he did not want to, stimulated him to an erection, and had sex with him. He didn't want to have sex with them; he was forced to—that's rape.[3]

The line between what is sexual assault and what is rape can be a blurry one for prosecutors, especially when the victim is a male. A letter posted anonymously to the Massachusetts Institute of Technology student newspaper, *The Tech*, claims it was a case of rape, but does not provide many details. Regardless, the student claims it was a case of rape:

I've been RAPED! It's a horrible thing to hear from someone you know, from someone you care about. It's a horrible thing to say to anyone, to your mother or father, to your best friend, *to yourself.*
"*I've been RAPED!*"
There! I said it!
That's right, I was raped. It happened in a fraternity. It happened right in my own bed; a place I considered safe. *I was raped by my girlfriend right in my own bed!* I knew what they were going to say:
"You shouldn't have let her get you drunk," or "You should have told her to go home," or "You should have just stopped it."

Oh, I tried not to give in to her pleading. I tried not to let her manipulate my mind. But she played on all my male insecurities and all my personal weaknesses. She was good at that. (She even threatened to start a rumor about the size of my masculinity.)

I told my friends what happened. . . . Most of them laughed at me or turned away in disbelief. Some of them even asked me if I enjoyed it! Some fraternity brothers they turned out to be! But, I suppose I should have expected it. Who is going to believe that the *man* got raped, right? . . .

But it does happen! Most rapes do not involve excessive force. So why can't a woman rape a man? Women talk about men overpowering them. The fact is that a woman can also overpower a man! Maybe she won't hit him or throw him across the room, but she might manipulate him emotionally or threaten him with slander. In many cases men give into these ploys and are coerced into doing things sexually that they may not want to do.[4]

Alexis Williams has a master's degree in Public Health at Emory University, and writes sexual advice columns for websites. In one column, she answers the question as well as anyone, in plain language about the most common questions—How can a man be raped if he is truly in fear? How could an erection be possible?

Men can, and are, raped by women. Though there are many backwards ass states in which a woman cannot be convicted of raping a man due to how rape is defined in that state. . . . This is related, in part, to two misconceptions. The first is that men always want sex and women don't have to force themselves. The second is that men must be aroused to have an erection. Both of these myths are wrong, wrong, wrong.

You are correct when you say that erections can be caused by anxiety. They also occur for no reason at all. . . . Most often erections are caused by sexual stimulation. And no—arousal and stimulation are not the same thing. Stimulation is a physical response to a stimulus. When someone steps on your toe, the stimulation you feel is pain and there is nothing you can do about that. If a woman performs oral sex on a man without his consent (which is rape) he can have an erection as a result. It does not mean that he is aroused. . . . So a man can be physically stimulated—without feeling aroused—causing an erection. He can be scared and intimidated into one, especially if the person is older or an authority figure and he can be forced into having intercourse. Forcing a man into oral or anal sex is also a form of rape, although these acts may not fall under legal definitions of rape. . . .

Unfortunately, these violations are not taken seriously because of this misguided idea that males always want sex. The trauma these boys and men face is very real and very serious. And it is an issue that deserves a lot more attention, discussion, and prevention than it is currently receiving.[5]

In the *Archives of Sexual Behavior*, pioneering medical researchers Philip Sarrel, MD, and William H. Masters, MD, flatly state the case for arousal even in terrifying situations: "The belief that it is impossible for males to respond sexually when subjected to sexual molestation by women is contradicted. Previous research indicating that male sexual response can occur in a variety of emotional states, including anger and terror, are corroborated."[6]

So, what are the facts? Does it really happen, and how often?

The Data

Prior to 1982, according to Sarrel and Masters, no research had ever been conducted, asking men if they had been the victims of sexual assault by women.[7]

We now turn to national crime statistics and things get a bit murky. According to the 1997 National Crime Victimization Survey (NCVS), 9 percent of the victims of rape and sexual assault are male.[8]

These figures do, however, include males who raped other males. Digging a little deeper into the Justice Department survey figures, we find that females committed 2 percent of all single-offender rapes and sexual assaults, and 6 percent of all multiple-offender rapes and sexual assaults. This still does not tell us, though, how many and what percentage were adult female-to-adult male cases nor how many were female against female.

Furthermore, the NCVS, though quite large, at 50,000 households, is much like the census. It is *not confidential*. It goes to households, not individuals. It asks questions about all types of crime, burglary, and so on. Consistently on this issue, for example, of all types of intimate partner violence surveys that are confidential (either by telephone, or even better, self-administered confidential surveys), the results compared to the NCVS show a much higher total of this more intimate type of crime.

We can now look to a different kind of crime reporting, which the Bureau of Justice Statistics helpfully explains: "The National Incident-Based Reporting System (NIBRS) represents the next generation of crime data from law enforcement agencies. It is designed to replace the nearly 70-year-old UCR program that compiles aggregate data on eight crimes. Rather than relying on a narrow group of 8 Index offenses, which are meant to convey the overall crime situation, NIBRS collects information on 57 types of crimes."

The Uniform Crime Report (UCR) is a measure of reported crimes by law enforcement agencies; thus, it is quite different from the Justice Department's general population survey. Interestingly, in the most recent report from the first three states participating in this new system (representing about 3 percent of the U.S. population), the results were somewhat surprising—About 10 percent of the rapes in the three states did not conform to the UCR definition of forcible rape—as the victims were male (8.7% of rapes), the victim and offender were both female (0.8%), or the victim was male and the offender was female (0.2%).[9]

A further analysis of the new system of crime reporting, now with 12 states participating, found an increase in the number of males being raped—up to 14 percent of the total instead of just 10 percent: "Nearly all of the offenders in sexual assaults reported to law enforcement were male (96%). Female offenders were most common in assaults against victims under age 6. For these youngest victims, 12% of offenders were females, compared with 6% for victims ages 6 through 12, and 3% for victims ages 12 through 17. Overall, 6% of the offenders who sexually assaulted juveniles were female compared with just 1% of the female offenders who sexually assaulted adults."[10]

We can now turn to other types of instruments that measure this type of crime; these include surveys that are confidential and focus on a particular area, rather than all types of crime.

- About three percent of American men—a total of 2.78 million men—have experienced an attempted or completed rape in their lifetime according to the 1998 Prevalence, Incidence and Consequences of Violence Against Women study (More commonly known as the Violence Against Women Survey).[11]

This survey, funded by the Justice Department, and the Centers for Disease Control and Prevention (CDC), but using a somewhat different methodology that traditionally results in higher total numbers of crime victims than the general crime survey (NCVS), found that, "Using a definition of rape that includes completed or *attempted* (emphasis added) forced vaginal, oral and anal sex, the survey found 7.7 percent of surveyed women and 0.3 percent of surveyed men being raped by a current or former intimate partner at some time in their lifetime."[12]

However, this Violence Against Women Survey only measured intimate partner violence, stranger rapes were not measured.

As prosecutor Jon Love noted, and all the other prosecutors and law enforcement officials we have talked with agreed, men are much less likely to report being raped, whether by a man or a woman. Rape crisis counselors estimate that while only one in 50 raped women report the crime to the police, the rates of under-reporting by men are assumed to be even higher.

Writing in the journal *Sex Roles: A Journal of Research*, authors Nathan W. Pino and Robert F. Meier sum up the current thinking on this issue:

We might expect that the reasons for male victim rape reporting would parallel those for women, but we should acknowledge the possibility that different forces may operate with males. Male rape is one of the least discussed crimes in our society (Groth and Burgess, 1980). . . . In addition, male victims may experience being raped as even more humiliating than female victims. As with female victims (Adler, 1992; Groth and Burgess, 1980), the emotional trauma experienced by raped males can generate confusion and inhibit reporting. A majority of males attempt to control their emotional reactions, reflecting a gender role expectation that it is unmanly for men to express emotion, even when the man is under a great deal of physical or emotional distress (Kaufman et al., 1980). Because reports of male rape are statistically rare male victims experience the additional trauma of making it difficult to identify with other male victims. Research has also shown that males are more likely to be victims of multiple assailants, to sustain more physical trauma, and to be held captive longer than female victims (Kaufman et al., 1980). Such feelings virtually guarantee low rape reporting rates. Reporting a rape to the police is at least as stressful for men as women (Groth and Burgess, 1980), but the extent to which victims subscribe to a male ethic of self-reliance, reporting may be further depressed. As in nonsexual areas of their lives, men are generally expected to defend themselves against threats (Finklehor, 1984, pp. 156–157). Along with this idea is the implicit belief that rape is synonymous with the loss of masculinity (Groth and Burgess, 1980; Adler, 1992). For these reasons, there may be substantial risk to the male rape victim's self-concept in reporting this crime.[13]

In *The Journal of Sex Research*, one study did find that actual physical violence used by women against men to force sexual intercourse was reported half as frequently:

Female against Male: 1.4%
Male against Female: 2.7%[14]

If this study is accurate, can we safely say that slightly more than 1 percent of men over a lifetime have been raped by a woman?

A large-scale survey of more than 3,000 Los Angeles area men and women, conducted in 1987, defined sexual assault as being forced or pressured to have sexual contact. Seven percent of the men said they had been victims and 2 percent reported being threatened with a weapon. However, this study did not distinguish between male and female perpetrators.[15]

A University of South Dakota survey of 268 men found that 16 percent reported at least one incident of a forced sexual experience in their lifetime. Nine percent of the men had been victims since becoming college students. Men in this study were actually somewhat *more likely* than women to say they had forced sex while on a date. Ten percent were physically forced to have intercourse with the perpetrator. The study is a little unclear, but the article indicates that these perpetrators were women rather than men.[16]

Looking at the numbers, rather than the percentages in the survey, 21 men out of the 268 reported physically forced intercourse. Another college survey of 507 males found that 2.2 percent had been the victims of violent sexual physical coercion.[17]

Does this mean that somewhere between 2 percent and 10 percent of college-age men have been raped by women? Although nearly 1,000 college-age men were surveyed in these two studies, such a blanket statement seems premature. They are an important indicator, however, and it does seem to show that, far from being an extremely rare occurrence, rape of men by women does occur with greater frequency than is most often assumed. More research is needed, with specific questions about the type of attack and what kinds of force were used.

We do have some confirmation from a much larger survey of nearly 2,500 men with the median age of 40. Of these, 3 percent reported having nonconsensual sex as an adult. About half reported that the non-consensual sex was with a woman. Since this apparently is the largest survey ever done of adult men about nonconsensual sex and not limited just to college-age respondents, we should take a close look at the results, as reported in *The British Medical Journal*.[18]

Since nearly 1.5 percent of the men over a lifetime reported nonconsensual sex with an adult woman, does that mean that they were raped? It depends, once again, on how rape is defined. The researchers listed a number of choices for the respondents, from having their or the perpetrator's genitals touched to even being made to urinate on the perpetrator.

It is a little easier to analyze the results if we report the numbers rather than the percentages. Thirty-two men reported nonconsensual adult sex, with women as the perpetrators. Of these, 1 reported anal penetration and 14 reported being made to have intercourse.

To put it another way, this large survey found that, over a lifetime, *less than* 1 percent of men report forced anal or vaginal intercourse with an adult woman. Or, 15 men out of 2,474 who agreed to answer the confidential computerized questionnaire. Interestingly, there was a slightly higher number of men who reported any nonconsensual adult sex if the researcher was a male, even though the actual answers were recorded in private.

Another way of examining the question of how frequently rape of men by adult women occurs is to examine women raping women. Researcher Claire Renzetti has been a pioneer in examining abuse of all types in lesbian relationships. Forty-eight percent of the respondents in a survey she helped conduct said they had experienced sexual abuse in their relationships and had experienced forced sex, with 16 percent saying it was forced upon them frequently. Four percent of the respondents had suffered a gun or knife being inserted in their vagina.[19]

Does this mean that lesbians are more likely to rape other lesbians than it is for a woman to rape a man? Possibly.

Stranger rape of women by women is no doubt less common than intimate partner rape, but even that does occur. In Seattle, Bridget Latrice Brown, 23, pleaded guilty to second-degree rape and third-degree robbery in a 1997 attack. According to King County court reports, Brown knocked on the victim's door, saying she was selling magazines. The victim did not want to buy anything, but let Brown in to use the telephone. Brown then brandished a knife, tied the woman up, and sexually assaulted her.[20]

Given the lack of details about the offender–victim relationship in many crime survey instruments, and the underreporting reflected even more strongly by male victims in actual reported crime statistics, the authors conclude that we do not know nearly as much as we should about the actual rate of adult male rape by adult females. This however, is likely to change in the future.

There is no question that the highly publicized cases in recent years of adult females raping boys (the Mary Kay Letourneau case, for example, in which the former school teacher was imprisoned for having sex with a 14-year-old boy) have spurred law enforcement and general public attention to this crime as well as new research.

It is likely that this book, as well as probable future highly publicized events, will spur further research and analysis of male rape by adult women. Using a strict definition of rape as *forced* vaginal or anal intercourse, however, the truth is that despite a careful review of the available research, we cannot say with *certainty* just how often it occurs.

Since this book is apparently the first to offer a comprehensive examination of the available research on forced vaginal and anal rape by adult women against adult men, however, we would be remiss if we did not come to some firm conclusions:

- *A conservative estimate is that over an average lifetime, at least 1 percent of adult men have been rape victims of adult women. Considering the likelihood of under-reporting either to law enforcement, counselors, or researchers, the percentage could be as high as 5 percent.*
- Given the population in the United States of adult men, this means that approximately 585,000 to 2,929,663 are the victims of vaginal or anal rape by adult women over a lifetime.
- On an annual basis, between 5,859 and 146,483 adult women rape adult men.

This may be a startling figure to some, but notice how rape is defined, as "forced penetration."

The New Definition of Rape

In 2011, three events took place that will likely change the sexual landscape in the United States.

In April 2011, the U.S. Department of Education issued a directive to all institutions of higher learning that receive any type of federal funds. The directive was issued without prior notice or opportunity for public comment: "[I]n order for a school's grievance procedures to be consistent with Title IX standards, the school *must* (emphasis added) use a preponderance of the evidence standard (i.e., *it is more likely than not* that sexual harassment or violence occurred)."

Discussion of this directive in which schools could lose federal funds if they fail to follow this policy is reserved for our final chapter.

The second event in October 2011 was even more groundbreaking— the Federal Bureau of Investigation (FBI) changed the definition of what rape is. The previous definition had been in place for 80 years: "The carnal knowledge of a female forcibly and against her will."

The U.S. Justice Department and the FBI, under the direction of the Uniform Crime Report Subcommittee, has changed that definition to: "Penetration, *no matter how slight* (emphasis added), of the vagina or anus with any body part or object, or oral penetration by a sex organ of another person, *without the consent of the victim* (emphasis added)."

The third event occurred in November 2011, the release of the Centers for Disease Control and Prevention, National Intimate Partner and Sexual Violence Survey. This survey also created a new definition of rape by the federal government—not only forced or attempted forced penetration, but also "alcohol/drug facilitated completed penetration."

Thus, the CDC declared: "Nearly 1 in 5 women (18.3%) and 1 in 71 men (1.4%) in the United States have been raped at some time in their lives, including completed forced penetration, attempted forced penetration, or alcohol/drug facilitated completed penetration."[21]

The report made front-page news across the country and the details, as usual, were left in the dust, with most headlines carrying the news that one in five women have been raped.

Criticism and Analysis of the CDC Survey

The following contains part of a letter sent and prepared by Stop Abusive and Violent Environments or SAVE (at the time, I was a board member of this organization, so it was delivered under my signature, but I am no longer with this group) to the CDC director in charge of this survey and we include here a considerable part of the CDC response to that letter.

Questions Are Raised about the Definition

The SAVE letter contends that the survey artificially inflates the number of female rape victims in two ways:

1. Counts a rape *attempt* the same as the actual commission of the act. We know of no area of criminal law where an attempt is afforded the same legal status as the actual crime. While it is legitimate to assess rape attempts, such attempts should not be subsumed within the category of rapes.

2. Counts alcohol/drug facilitated completed penetration as a form of rape.

The SAVE letter contends that the NISVS does not account for situations in which a couple indulges in alcohol or drugs and then engages in sexual relations, for example, after a New Year's Eve party. For the sake of clarity and accuracy, we show here the text of the actual questions from the survey:

When you were drunk, high, drugged, or passed out and unable to consent, how many people ever . . .

- had vaginal sex with you? By vaginal sex, we mean that (if female, a man or boy put his penis in your vagina) (if male, a woman or girl made you put your penis in her vagina)?
- (if male) made you perform anal sex, meaning that they made you put your penis into their anus?
- made you receive anal sex, meaning they put their penis into your anus?
- made you perform oral sex, meaning that they put their penis in your mouth or made you penetrate their vagina or anus with your mouth?
- made you receive oral sex, meaning that they put their mouth on your (if male: penis) (if female: vagina) or anus?

The SAVE letter asked the CDC to consider this scenario: "A woman invites a friend to her apartment for dinner. They consume two bottles of wine. Then, she invites him to her bedroom for sex." (The SAVE letter also included a similar scenario about a husband and wife.) "When asked, 'When you were drunk, high, drugged, or passed out and unable to consent, how many people ever . . . had vaginal sex with you?,' the woman can honestly answer 'yes.' So, the female initiator of sex becomes classified by the NISVS as a victim of rape.

"Upon reflection, one can identify many other scenarios in which the NISVS definition leads to a nonintuitive conclusion and an over-count of the number of rape victims.

"Of course, alcohol/drug-facilitated rape is a real problem in our society, and the issue is an important one to study. But, if CDC wishes to assess the prevalence of alcohol/drug-facilitated rape, it must also evaluate the timing of the consent and who the initiator of the action was. Furthermore, it must be not undermine current legal definitions of rape.

"In a time of shrinking social services, it is critical that true victims of rape receive priority for services and support. By defining rape broadly, the publicity surrounding the NISVS may lead to an increase in the number of persons inappropriately claiming to be victims of rape, thus diverting essential services from the real victims."[22]

The CDC Responds

The CDC responded in this manner to the questions raised by the letter composed by Stop Abusive and Violent Environments and sent under this author's signature:

> On the topic of inclusion of and classification alcohol and drug facilitated sexual violence, it seems there has been a misunderstanding of how these questions were framed and administered. We have gone to great lengths to ensure that respondents understand these two components-the use of substances and the inability to give consent-as part of the administration of these questions. . . . The term consent is included in the question as well as the narrative text that precedes these questions. The interviewers state, "Sometimes sex happens when a person is unable to consent or stop it from happening, because they were too drunk, high, drugged or passed out from alcohol, drugs, or medications. The scenario of consensual sex between a husband and wife after drinking at a New Year's Eve party would not meet the definition of what is included in this series of NISVS questions."[23]

Undercounts Male Victims

The SAVE letter contended,

> In . . . important ways, the NISVS undercounts the number of male victims.
>
>   Sexual Violence: Being Made to Penetrate Someone—The NISVS defines "being made to" as a person using "physical force or threats to physically harm you" (page 106). The far more common scenario is a woman who physically stimulates the man in an unwanted manner to the point of sexual arousal. But the NISVS *excludes* this scenario from its definition of Being Made to Penetrate Someone.

These limited measures reduce the number of male victims relative to females; bias the study conclusions, influence public opinion, and may even serve to create a double-standard of justice.[24]

The CDC Responds

You also raise the issue of potential bias from the wording of the question for men in terms of being "made to" penetrate someone else creating consideration of coercion that does not exist for women. Adding the "made to" language for women *has merit* (emphasis added) and will be taken into consideration as we refine the instrument for future years of data collection. You also point out that NISVS measure of made to penetrate does not include a measure of unwanted physical stimulation to the point of arousal. This type of abusive sexual contact is captured in NISVS as unwanted sexual contact rather than made to penetrate, but, we continue to consider additions and modifications to further improve on our data collection and *may consider* (emphasis added) making this kind of victimization more clearly specified.[25]

It should also be noted that the definition does not include "envelopment" but only "penetration."

False Statements?

The SAVE letter claims that the NISVS report contains a number of statements that are "One-sided, or have little or no basis in scientific fact."

The CDC report contains this statement: "[W]omen are heavily affected by sexual violence, stalking and intimate partner violence" (p. 83). The SAVE letter contended that "This statement is one-sided, misleading, and false, since the NISVS demonstrates men are more 'heavily affected' by physical violence, coercive violence, and reproductive control than women."

The CDC replied, and flatly rejected this contention: "The statement that women are more heavily affected by these issues refers to the differences observed in the forms, severity and impact of violence for women and is accurate."[26]

The CDC response letter does not offer any references or support for their statement that women are more "heavily affected," but in any case, it is certainly an unsupported statement since the survey did not measure sex differences in regards to the impact of behaviors or actions.

In other words, for the CDC to fully support this statement, they would need to include questions about "forms, severity and impact" within this particular survey. To rely on unnamed other research in an important government document may or may not be false, but it is certainly misleading. This survey is unique, as questions were asked about a set of behaviors about which such questions had never before been asked in a large nationally representative sample survey.

What evidence is there to support the contention that one sex is more heavily affected than the other by violence, either sexual violence or other forms of violence? Research in this area is, at the current time, quite limited, mainly because men are often left out as subjects. Is it not more likely that both sexes are negatively affected? Is it true, for example, that a gay male who is raped by another man suffers less than a heterosexual male who is forcibly raped by another man? I would contend that there would be very little or no difference. Others might contend there would be a difference, but the truth is, we don't know. The variable is the extent, nature, and consequences of such violence, and that is connected more concretely to individual circumstances rather than gender. To put it in another context, did Ron Varga of Spokane suffer less than a woman would have, under the same set of circumstances?

The SAVE letter to the CDC also had two other criticisms: "Media messages that 'reinforce negative stereotypes about masculinity' (p. 89)—This statement is demeaning and insulting, and should be removed. . . . and that create a social climate that *condones* sexual violence, stalking, and intimate partner violence (p. 89)—This unsupported—and unsupportable—statement verges on the absurd."[27]

The CDC did not directly reply to these two criticisms in their reply letter, except to say that, "We know from other research that social structures and social norms are important areas for primary prevention activities in terms of supporting women and men in rejecting violence as acceptable."[28]

The CDC explanation is fine in terms of wanting to support both women and men in rejecting violence as acceptable, but that is not what the report said; it focused only on inhibiting such behaviors in men, not women. In other words, the report focused only on media messages that deal with masculinity, not with media messages that support female misbehavior or even violence against men. It would take another media matters book in itself to explore and examine media images and make some sort of determination as to which gender fares worse. In terms of just television commercials condoning violence against intimate partners, however, we can certainly conclude that there are more instances where the victim is a man than a woman. To give but one example (since it was a 2011 Super Bowl commercial, it was widely seen), Pepsi showed a woman violently shoving her boyfriend's or husband's face into a plate of food and then throwing a can at him. It may be supposed that organizations such as the National Coalition Against Domestic Violence would launch a protest campaign against such a national commercial in such a prime time spot if it was a woman who was treated in such a violent manner, but they were silent when the victim was a man. It apparently is just humorous when it happens to a man, and any men who complain (the National Coalition For Men did) are often dismissed as whining males. Certainly, it is true that such organizations' complaints are not the subject of any news media coverage, whereas if the National Organization for Women or even the National Coalition Against Domestic Violence made a similar complaint on the same type of subject, there is high degree of likelihood that their complaint would receive some news media coverage or at least coverage, say, in the blogosphere of websites such as *The Huffington Post*.

The reader may recall that men were somewhat more revealing about nonconsensual sex experiences in the previously mentioned *British Medical Journal* study when the interviewer was male, compared to female interviewers. Thus, either the CDC was not aware of this research or if aware, chose to ignore it. We will not assume that this is simply a case of verifiable sexism in choosing only female interviewers, despite the hiring bias. There is some evidence to suggest that, in a telephone interview survey, people are more likely to respond and complete a survey if only female interviewers are used. This is perhaps why the CDC chose only females, and indeed, they indicated this is the reason they chose this methodology. However, answering questions about which soap is used, in a typical marketing survey, is far different and perhaps contraindicated in a survey about sexual behaviors.

The data that the CDC reports in the NISVS is extremely valuable in terms of what was discovered, even discounting the fact that only female interviewers were used to conduct it, but what is disturbing is how ideological bias flavored conclusions and presentation of the data in the reports' summary statements. Up until this report, the CDC could be relied upon to present such data in an unbiased, nonsexist manner; now, with this report, summary statements must be examined as possibly suspect. The genesis and basis for this creeping ideology finding its way into even the formerly purely scientific halls of the CDC is explored a bit further in this chapter and in the concluding chapter.

Table 1.1   NISVS Data on Male Sexual Victimization

	Lifetime		12 month	
Rape (2)	*	*	*	*
Other Sexual Violence	8.0	9,050,000	2.5	2,793,000
Made to penetrate	2.2	2,442,000	0.5	586,000
Sexual coercion(3)	4.2	4,744,000	1.0	1,143,000
Unwanted sexual contact(4)	2.6	2,999,000	0.9	1,031,000
Non-contact unwanted sexual experiences(5)	2.7	3,049,000	0.8	882,000

Source: M. C. Black, K. C. Basile, M. J. Breiding, S. G. Smith, M. L. Walters, M. T. Merrick, J. Chen, and M. R. Stevens, *The National Intimate Partner and Sexual Violence Survey (NISVS): 2010 Summary Report*, National Center for Injury Prevention and Control, Centers for Disease Control and Prevention.

Despite these deficiencies and problems, the CDC report does provide some interesting data for our subject here in terms of *sexual assaults against men*, as Table 1.1 attests.

As the table shows, being rounded to the nearest thousand, (2) Includes completed forced penetration, attempted forced penetration, and completed alcohol/drug-facilitated rape, (3) Pressured in a nonphysical way (includes, for example, threatening to end the relationship, using influence or authority), (4) Includes unwanted kissing in a sexual way, fondling, or grabbing sexual body parts, (5) Includes, for example, exposing sexual body parts, being made to look at or participate in sexual photos or movies, harassed in a public place in a way that felt unsafe.

The CDC also reported these results from the survey for *women*:

Sexual Violence by an Intimate Partner—Prevalence among Women

Nearly 1 out of 10 women in the United States (9.4% or approximately 11.1 million) has been raped by an intimate partner in her lifetime. More specifically, 6.6 percent of women reported completed forced penetration by an intimate partner, 2.5 percent reported attempted forced penetration, and 3.4 percent reported alcohol or drug-facilitated rape. Approximately one in six women (16.9% or nearly 19 million) has experienced sexual violence other than rape by an intimate partner in her lifetime; this includes sexual coercion (9.8%), unwanted sexual contact (6.4%), and noncontact unwanted sexual experiences (7.8%).

In the 12 months prior to taking the survey, 0.6 percent or an estimated 686,000 women in the United States indicated that they were raped by an intimate partner, and 2.3 percent or an estimated 2.7 million women experienced other forms of sexual violence by an intimate partner.

Prevalence among Men

Too few men reported rape by an intimate partner to produce reliable prevalence estimates. Approximately 1 in 12 men in the United States (8.0% or approximately 9 million) has experienced sexual violence other than rape by an intimate partner in his lifetime. This includes being made to penetrate an intimate partner (2.2%), sexual coercion (4.2%), unwanted sexual contact (2.6%), and noncontact unwanted sexual experiences (2.7%). In the 12 months prior to taking the survey, 2.5 percent or nearly *2.8 million men experienced sexual violence other than rape by an intimate partner.*[29]

To summarize, 1 in 6 women and 1 in 12 men over a lifetime experienced sexual violence other than rape. The CDC did not, however, differentiate sexual violence initiated by women and that initiated by men against either sex.

The New FBI Definition of Rape

The new definition does not change the law immediately, it will— eventually. What it does change immediately is the reporting requirements of the law enforcement agencies that send information to the Justice Department. This information, in turn, is collated by the department and then makes up the annual Uniform Crime Report. This document is the standard by which all crime in the United States is measured.

In a conference call in January 2012, which I listened to, representatives from the Justice Department, law enforcement officials, and Feminist Majority (more on their participation and direction in this and our final chapter), said that it would take about two years for this new definition to be assimilated by the reporting agencies and then be reflected in the Uniform Crime Report.

We can then expect a huge increase in the reported instances of the crime of rape, in about 2014, even while other crimes (mainly due to the age of population and other factors) remain stable or are in decline. Thus, a new kind of "rape crisis" will have been created—with crime figures to prove it—and there will, no doubt, be increased pressure to change laws to meet the new "epidemic."

The previous definition, "The carnal knowledge of a female forcibly and against her will," has deficiencies, of course—male rape by this definition does not exist. What "carnal knowledge" is or is not has been open to legal interpretation by law enforcement agencies and in the courts, which indeed was part of the problem with the old definition.

The new definition, "Penetration, *no matter how slight*, of the vagina or anus with any body part or object, or oral penetration by a sex organ of another person, without the consent of the victim," is much broader. *Force is no longer necessary to classify such conduct as rape.*

Has she/he had a drink or two of alcohol or used a drug? Then, they are "incapable of consent" even if she/he voluntarily became inebriated.

Los Angeles attorney Marc Angelucci says,

> Think about what the new definition of rape means. Every exploratory hands-on teenager in the back seat of a car or on a sofa in the parents' basement is now at risk of being branded a rapist. They kiss. His hand touches ("penetration, no matter how slight, of the vagina or anus with any body part"). She does nothing ("without the consent" means he has the burden to get consent; she doesn't have to express lack of consent). He stops touching. Too late. The hand committed rape and the only question is whether she will press charges. *By changing the definition at the FBI data collection level, all jurisdictions will come under pressure to change their underlying statutes to make the crime fit the Federal definition.*[30]

Angelucci and other attorneys I have contacted remind us that in the FBI definition, the key is "without consent" and alcohol is not even mentioned. This is a huge inversion from "against her will." "Against her will" indicates a need for her to give some clue that his advances are unwelcome and give her a chance to desist his advances. "Without consent" means that he needs something affirmative from her and *he is a rapist if he does not have that affirmative proof of consent.*

Does this mean that every sexual event between adults (married or not, as marital rape can also be charged) will now require, as protection against a rape or sexual assault charge, a signed sexual conduct agreement contract?

Another View of the New Definition

In an email correspondence, I asked the directors of the leading male sexual victim organization MaleSurvivor, what they thought of the big change:

> Our major concern is that the definition was limited to females being victims. The new definition definitely makes it possible for the definition to include male rape and sexual assault victims, which is a major step forward. . . . I believe if someone is drunk or drugged, whether by their own choosing or not, in my mind they are not capable of giving consent. I see it as a major shift in government policy and as a strong message to our society that it is time to start protecting people who are unable to protect themselves. And it is time for men and women who are being sexual to be held accountable and responsible for healthy sexual behaviors that respect the rights of the partners and the need to give consent as a part of those experiences.
>
> After the committee at the FBI determined the new definition we issued the statement below. No one contacted us directly prior to the committee's report to the director. I did send the statement below to the director after the committee made its recommendation.
>
> My understanding is that the definition will change reporting more than enforcement since the crimes previously was prosecuted as sexual assault will now be included in reporting as rape.[31]
>
> —Howard Fradkin, PhD

Although definitions used for reporting purposes such as this do not limit investigation of sexual assault, it is important to acknowledge the reality that rape victimization and perpetration are not limited by gender. This removal of gender bias from the FBI's rape definition will help men who have been raped by helping to remove the false argument "Men can't be raped" from the preconceptions that our society accepts. Inclusion of male victims in reporting will encourage boys and men to report the sexual crime committed against them.[32]

—Ken Followell, President, MaleSurvior

Prime Movers behind the Change

It was a fictional character in the novel by Marilyn French, *The Women's Room*, who declared that, "All men are rapists." A fictional assertion and one that in truth neither celebrated feminists Andrea Dworkin or Catharine MacKinnon ever stated—nor has either declared that "all sex is rape." Here are a few quotes that *are* accurate:

Quotes by Andrea Dworkin[33]

"Intercourse as an act often expresses the power men have over women."
"Seduction is often difficult to distinguish from rape. In seduction, the rapist often bothers to buy a bottle of wine."

Quotes by Catharine MacKinnon

"Politically, I call it rape whenever a woman has sex and feels violated."[34]
"Men who are in prison for rape think it's the dumbest thing that ever happened . . . It isn't just a miscarriage of justice; they were put in jail for something very little different from what most men do most of the time and call it sex. The only difference is they got caught. That view is non-remorseful and not rehabilitative. It may also be true."[35]

There is also this exchange from a PBS television interview program:

Mr. Wattenberg: Okay. So what is, then, your definition of rape? Does this—is this always a violent confrontation with a man subordinating a woman against her will? Is that what we're talking about?
Ms. MacKinnon: That's generally what people think of it as. I think, though, there are forms of force that involve authority, power, where something can be rape, but it isn't always violent at that moment. But there's always an element of force and domination going on in it and there is—in which a sexual interaction is coerced without the person who is having it wanting to have the sex.[36]

Camille Paglia in *Vamps and Tramps* has an altogether different view:

What began as a useful sensitization of police officers, prosecutors and judges to the claims of authentic rape victims turned into a hallucinatory overextension of the definition of rape to cover every unpleasant or embarrassing sexual encounter. Rape became the crime of crimes, overshadowing all the wars, massacres, and disasters of world history. The feminist obsession with rape as a symbol of male–female relations is irrational and delusional. From the perspective of the future, this period in America will look like a reign of mass psychosis, like that of the Salem witch trials. Rape cannot be understood in isolation from general criminology, which most feminists have not bothered to study. . . . The fantastic fetishism of rape by mainstream and anti-porn feminists has in the end trivialized rape, impugned women's credibility, and reduced the sympathy we should feel for legitimate victims of violent sexual assault.[37]

Are the new definitions of rape, both in the CDC survey and the FBI definition, in which inebriation defines nonconsensual and force is no longer needed to define rape, a victorious culmination of the Dworkian–MacKinnon view of the world? Did they or the supporters of this gender–feminist worldview, have in reality, anything to do with it?

In January 2012, the Justice Department held a conference call regarding their new definition. Organized in part by that department and also held under the auspices of the White House Council for Women (there is no White House Council for Men—and calls for its creation have fallen on deaf ears). In the call which I listened in on (comments or participation by noninvited guests were limited to only email questions), it was proudly noted by several participants that "many victim advocate groups" were solicited for their views on the definition, prior to it being ratified.

MaleSurvivor must be considered one of the leading anti-rape/sexual assault organizations for men. Dr. Fradkin's statement is telling: "No one contacted us directly prior to the committee's report to the director."[38] Present on the call however, as an honored guest, and acknowledged by others as a leading instigator of this change was a representative of Feminist Majority.

This organization heralded the change with a press release, announcing: "We Did It: Feminist Majority Foundation Celebrates FBI Approval of New Rape Definition—FBI Director's Action Follows Extensive Campaign By Women's Rights Supporters."

"Updating the FBI Uniform Crime Report definition of rape is a big win for women," said Eleanor Smeal, president of Feminist Majority Foundation. "We appreciate the support for this change from the Obama Administration, led by Vice President Joe Biden and by Lynn Rosenthal, White House Advisor on Violence Against Women, and Hon. Susan B. Carbon, director of the Office on Violence Against Women in the Department of Justice, as well as the FBI." The White House today announced that FBI Director Robert Mueller has approved the change recommended by several committees of the FBI's Criminal Justice Information Service.[39]

On the call, the Feminist Majority representative said, "Well, we know that two-thirds of the rapes on campus are because of inebriation."

So, every drunken hook-up on campus is a case of rape? Well, it appears so. If you are drunk, you are incapable of consent, and without consent, it is rape, if the "victim" decides to make it so, the morning after, or whenever.

The Feminist Majority website also applauded Vice President Joe Biden's statements on the issue: "But whether someone is drunk or sober doesn't matter. As Biden put it, 'Look folks—rape is rape is rape.' . . . That's one message that Biden hit hard: 'Look guys—no matter what a girl does, no matter how she's dressed, no matter how much she's had to drink, it's never, never, never, never OK to touch her without her consent. This doesn't make you a man. It makes you a coward.' "[40]

Is a touch rape? Apparently so. In the world of Biden, the Feminist Majority, and now, the FBI, "consent" seems to be the operative word. So, what is that, by their definition?

Consent

If consent is not obtained prior to each act of sexual behavior (from kissing leading up to intercourse), a student risks violation of the Vassar College Sexual Misconduct Policy. . . .

Consent Is:
A voluntary, sober, imaginative, enthusiastic, creative, wanted, informed, mutual, honest, and verbal agreement.

- An active agreement: Consent cannot be coerced
- A process, which must be asked for every step of the way; if you want to move to the next level of sexual intimacy, just ask
- Never implied and cannot be assumed.[41]

This college's definition is typical and certainly not exclusive to Vassar. Look for this definition at a college near you (where one can be brought up on charges of sexual assault or rape under the college's own rules, not those of a court of law, as we explore in our final chapter) and soon in your state's law or interpretations in the court of what is meant by consent.

Dr. Ava Cadell is a private therapist who has gained a national reputation as a sex advice expert and appeared on numerous national television shows. She strongly advises that every couple sign a consent to have sexual relations form. Her website lists a number of reasons for such a signed document, but one statement did catch my eye: "The Sexual Consent Form can protect men from manipulative women who may bring false charges of sexual misconduct for financial gain. Remember that even men who have no assets need to protect themselves from false accusations because they can lose everything including their property, freedom, and their reputation until found innocent."[42] Dr. Cadell helpfully provides such a form on her website.

Well, it is only one page long and could probably be folded and kept in a man's wallet along with the condom.

Camille Paglia again:

> Even the most morbid of the rape ranters have a childlike faith in the perfectibility of the universe, which they see as blighted solely by nasty men. They simplistically project outward onto a mythical patriarchy their own inner conflicts and moral ambiguities. . . . Feminism has constructed a spectral sexual hell that these girls inhabited; it was their entire cultural world, a godless new religion of fury and fanaticism. . . . It produces young women unable to foresee trouble or to survive sexual misadventure or even raunchy language with crying to authority figures for help. A sense of privilege and entitlement, as well as ignorance of the dangers of life, has been institutionalized.[43]

Paglia was speaking about the college campus, but she correctly foresaw the institutionalization of these precepts and worldview in the broader society, and indeed, it has come to pass.

Consequences

Meanwhile, The National Center For Victims of Crime succinctly address some of the issues that male victims of rape face:

Case research suggests that males also commonly experience many of the reactions that females experience. Other problems facing males include an increased sense of vulnerability, damaged self-image and emotional distancing (Mezey & King, 1989). Male rape victims not only have to confront unsympathetic attitudes if they choose to press charges, they also often hear unsupportive statements from their friends, family and acquaintances (Brochman, 1991). . . .

It is not uncommon for a male rape victim to blame himself for the rape, believing that he in some way gave permission to the rapist (Brochman, 1991). Male rape victims suffer a similar fear that female rape victims face—that people will believe the myth that they may have enjoyed being raped. Some men may believe they were not raped or that they gave consent because they became sexually aroused, had an erection, or ejaculated during the sexual assault. These are normal, involuntary physiological reactions. It does not mean that the victim wanted to be raped or sexually assaulted, or that the survivor enjoyed the traumatic experience. . . .

Some assailants may try to get their victim to ejaculate because for the rapist, it symbolizes their complete sexual control over their victim's body. . . . This aspect of the attack is extremely stressful and confusing to the victim. In misidentifying ejaculation with orgasm, the victim may be bewildered by his physiological response during the sexual assault and, therefore, may be discouraged from reporting the assault for fear his sexuality may become suspect (Groth & Burgess, 1980). Another major concern facing male rape victims is society's belief that men should be able to protect themselves and, therefore, it is somehow their fault that they were raped.[44]

The consequences of male rape, according to the crime victims' center, are no less severe than they are for female victims:

- Rectal and anal tearing and abrasions which may require attention and be put them at risk for bacterial infections
- Potential HIV exposure; and exposure to other sexually transmitted diseases
- Loss of appetite; Nausea and/or stomachaches; Headaches
- Loss of memory and/or concentration; and/or Changes in sleep patterns

- Denial and/or Guilt
- Shame or humiliation
- Fear and a feeling of loss of control
- Loss of self-respect
- Flashbacks to the attack
- Anger and anxiety
- Retaliation fantasies (sometimes shocking the survivor with their graphic violence)
- Nervous or compulsive behavior.[45]

Werner Kierski writing in *Counseling and Psychotherapy Journal* found that it is often the case that psychologists and counselors fail to provide help to either female sexual abusers or male victims:

The issue is that female perpetrators of violence and their victims seldom receive proper help. Therefore cycles of violence and pain tend to remain unbroken: suffering and pain perpetuate themselves and trauma begets trauma. Organizers of the US based campaign to break the silence around sexual abuse of daughters by their mothers (Making Daughters Safe Again MDSA) say that mothers are capable of the same range of violence, hate and autonomous behavior as other human beings. MDSA points at the continuous failure of social workers and psychotherapists to detect understand and treat the victims and their perpetrators.

What is even more consternating is that although 81% of these victims are in therapy, only 3% have sufficient confidence in their psychotherapists to tell them about the abuse. Female sex offenders have lower rates in seeking help than male sex offenders. This again is a reflection of where the profession stands in relation to the problem.[46]

It is not the focus of this volume to deal in detail with the sexual abuse of children by men or women; it should be noted, however, that if we are concerned with the prevention of rape, one study found that as many as 60 percent of adult male rapists in the sample had been sexually molested during childhood by females, that in about 70 percent of the cases, the molesting person did so on more than one occasion, and that about 15 percent of male rapists had been molested during childhood by two or more females. Furthermore, in contrast to male molesters, where the preponderance of cases involve fondling or looking at the victim, female molesters were more than twice as likely as males to engage in actual penetration, cunnilingus, or fellatio. Mental health implications here seem straightforward.[47]

This anonymous post on a website must be treated for what it is, an unsubstantiated post on a website. My sense is that it does reflect the reality of the British writer. It is, however, instructive as to some of the issues male rape victims must deal with:

> Last time I saw her privately she turned up midway through the afternoon expecting sex. I declined. I was busy. She was outraged. I tried to calm her down by offering a cuppa and sitting and talking. She jumped me and pinned me on the couch. I'm no weakling. As a younger man I was one of the best javelin throwers in my country. But she was six or seven stone heavier than I. As it was over a hundred that day I was only wearing shorts and singlet. She had access to everything and made it clear she didn't mind *hurting* me. The only way out of the situation for me was violence for which I have zero capacity. I ended up complying. . . .
>
> Is that rape?
>
> I never really considered this until several years later when in counseling for childhood abuse. Interestingly counselors tell me that experience, another incident in my mid-twenties and one in my late teens are also rapes by their standard. . . .
>
> If the question is are some women willing to act in ways that constitute rape—assuming that forcing sex on somebody is rape—the answer must be yes. . . .
>
> One of my sisters found herself in a relationship that was on the skids. She concocted a plan. She offered herself up as designated driver at a particular event. Kept his glass full all night. She later had sex with him while he was basically comatose. Her aim had been to get pregnant. She succeeded. His family, very catholic, made him marry her. Intriguingly she brags about this openly to this day AND does it in his presence.[48]

The Law

In discussing male rape, The National Center for Victims of Crime also succinctly sums up the current state of confusion regarding rape laws and their application on behalf of male victims: "In some states, the word 'rape' is used only to define a forced act of vaginal sexual intercourse, and an act of forced anal intercourse is termed 'sodomy.'

In some states, the crime of sodomy also includes any oral sexual act. There are some states that now use gender-neutral terms to define acts of forced anal, vaginal or oral intercourse. Also, some states no longer use the terms 'rape' and 'sodomy,' rather all sex crimes are described as sexual assaults or criminal sexual conduct of various degrees depending on the use and amount of force or coercion on the part of the assailant."[49]

An article published as "Adult Male Sexual Assault in the Community" by Isely indicates that sodomy has recently been added to some state laws under the rape statute. Sodomy indicates that something, not necessarily a penis, penetrated the male victim's rectum. Isely reports one incident where a male was raped by a woman and upon calling a rape-crisis hotline and asking for assistance, the counselor told him that males could not be raped and then hung up on him. The victim called back three times and was hung up on by the counselor each time. The incident does show that male rape victims may frequently be mistreated by a system that is used to dealing only with female rape victims.[50] Researchers at Clark University have found that male victims of intimate partner violence are treated harshly by established domestic violence service providers, and many of these are co-associated with rape-crisis lines as well.[51] Thus, the male victim has very few places to turn to seek help. Help that is not available to males, but is available to women means that encouragement or assistance in reporting to police and prosecutors is less likely to occur.

Gender Bias in Sentencing

The sentencing disparity when a woman is prosecuted compared to sentences handed down for men is well documented by the Bureau of Justice Statistics and by other analysis. Women receive less prison time than men for all types of crime. The disparity in sentencing increases as the charges become more serious. Typical of such analysis is this one from the journal, *Women in Criminal Justice*: "*Selective chivalry* predicts that decision makers extend chivalry disproportionately to white females. *Differential discretion* suggests that disparity is most likely in informal decisions such as charge reduction rather than in formal decisions at final sentencing. Data for the analysis derived from 9,966 felony theft cases and 18,176 felony assault cases disposed in California. Gender disparity was evident in findings that females with no prior record were more likely than similar males to receive charge reductions, and this enhanced females' chances for probation. The only indication of selective chivalry was a greater tendency to change charges of assault to non-assault among white female defendants than among minority females. Pivotal decisions concerning charge reduction provided partial support for the notion of differential discretion."[52] One might assume that there has been a change since 1988, especially given the increased incarceration rates of women for crime in general. A more recent examination of the data in *Criminal Justice Policy Review* found no change: "Dramatic increases in the number of women incarcerated in state and federal prisons have led some researchers to conclude that differential sentencing of female offenders is a thing of the past. This study uses data on offenders convicted of felonies in Chicago, Miami, and Kansas City to address this issue. The authors find no evidence to support this 'gender neutrality' hypothesis. In all three jurisdictions, women face significantly lower odds of incarceration than do men. The results also reveal that the effect of race is conditioned by gender but the effect of gender, with only one exception, is not conditioned by race; harsher treatment of racial minorities is confined to men but more lenient treatment of women is found for both racial minorities and Whites."[53]

There is some limited analysis of whether or not gender bias in favor of women also exists when it comes to sexual assaults, which was examined in the journal *Feminist* and extends to criminal sex offenders. In *Feminist Criminology*, the authors conclude that there is significant sentencing bias: "The current research examines the utility of the evil woman hypothesis by examining sentencing discrepancies between male and female sex offenders. National Corrections Reporting Program data are used to identify sex offenders for the years 1994 to 2004 and the sentences they received for specific sex offenses. Statistical analyses reveal a significant difference in sentence length between men and women, but not in the expected direction. The evil woman hypothesis would assume women are sentenced more harshly, but data show men receive longer sentences for sex offenses than women. Support is provided for the chivalry hypothesis to explain immediate sentencing disparity."[54]

One case illustrates the likelihood of this as well as any other. The question that should be asked is whether a man who ripped off a woman's breast and ate it, would have received more than two and half years in prison. The BBC reported the sentencing result in Liverpool when a woman made such an attack:

> Amanda Monti, 24, flew into a rage when Geoffrey Jones, 37, rejected her advances at the end of a house party. . . . She pulled off his left testicle and tried to swallow it, before spitting it

out. . . . Monti admitted wounding and was jailed for two-and-a-half years. Sentencing Monti, Judge Charles James said it was a very serious injury and that Monti was not acting in self-defense. The court heard that Mr. Jones had ended his long-term but open relationship with Monti. . . . The pair remained on good terms. . . . She picked him up from a party and went for drinks at a friend's house where an argument ensued. In his statement Jones said she grabbed his genitals and pulled hard. He added: "That caused my underpants to come off and I found I was completely naked and in excruciating pain." The court heard that a friend saw Monti put Mr. Jones testicle into her mouth and try to swallow it. She choked and spat it back into her hand before the friend grabbed it and gave it back to Mr. Jones. Doctors were unable to re-attach the organ.[55]

Marital rape is another area in which we can expect that it is much more likely for the male to be prosecuted than the female. For example, in 1960, in the British divorce case of *Willan v. Willan*, Mr. Willan claimed that his wife used vile and offensive language and badgered him into having sexual intercourse, including pulling his hair, and rolling on top of him, until he consented. The court denied the divorce on grounds of cruelty, with the judge agreeing that had it been a wife who made a similar complaint, the decision would have been different: "In the case of a husband who has sexual intercourse it can only be said of him that what he does he does on purpose, and that sexual intercourse with his wife must be a voluntary act on his part."[56]

The War on Men

It may not seem germane at first glance to include here a brief discussion of the use of rape as tactic in war. Certainly, it has been used by combatants against women, but it has also been used against men and while information is difficult to obtain, there is a body of evidence that in warring African nations, currently, more men suffer from rape than do women. For our purposes here, however, it is instructive to note how the international community intentionally and deliberately ignores male rape. The investigative reporting of Will Storr in the UK's *Observer* and *Guardian* serves as a guide. Storr describes his visit to Uganda and other parts of war-torn Africa and he examined the research of Lara Stemple of the University of California's Health and Human Rights Law Project. She found many cases of sexual violence used against males all over the world. She also found systematic and intentional neglect of such victims by non-governmental organizations (NGOs) and international aid groups. Stemple reviewed more than 4,000 organizations that address sexual violence in wartime and found that only 3 percent even mentioned men as a concern of such violence, and even then, only as a small reference:

> (In Kampala, Uganda, the Refuge Law Project (RLP) British director, is Dr. Chris Dolan). Stemple's findings on the failure of aid agencies are no surprise to Dolan. "The organizations working on sexual and gender-based violence don't talk about it," he says. "It's systematically silenced." . . . As part of an attempt to correct this, the RLP produced a documentary in 2010 called *Gender Against Men*. When it was screened, Dolan says that attempts were made to stop him. "Were these attempts by people in well-known, international aid agencies?" I ask. "Yes," he replies. . . . "There's a fear among them that this is a zero-sum game; that there's a pre-defined cake and if you start talking about men, you're going to somehow eat a chunk of this cake that's taken them a long time to bake."
>
> When I contact Stemple by email, she describes a "constant drum beat that women are *the* rape victims" and a milieu in which men are treated as a "monolithic perpetrator class."
>
> "International human rights law leaves out men in nearly all instruments designed to address sexual violence," she continues. "The UN Security Council Resolution 1325 in 2000 treats wartime sexual violence as something that only impacts on women and girls . . . Secretary of State Hillary Clinton recently announced $44 million to implement this resolution. Because of its entirely exclusive focus on female victims, it seems unlikely that any of these new funds will reach the thousands of men and boys who suffer from this kind of abuse. Ignoring male rape not only neglects men, it also harms women by reinforcing a viewpoint that equates 'female' with 'victim', thus hampering our ability to see women as strong and empowered. In the same way, silence about male victims reinforces unhealthy expectations about men and their supposed invulnerability."[57]

The intentional and deliberate silence enforced by international aid agencies in this area is, unfortunately, no surprise. Stemple's comments are on point in our particular discussion here of adult female rape of adult men. The neglect of male rape victims in all its various permutations is perhaps particularly pernicious when it comes to prison rape or war rape, but the effects of that neglect are the same when it comes to male victims of female rape and other forms of this type of crime.

The increased willingness of prosecutors in recent years to make cases against adult females who abuse boys may mean that we will see increased prosecutions against adult women for sexual assaults against adult men, though a charge of rape is likely to remain rare.

What is unlikely to remain rare, and in fact will definitely increase, are false allegations of rape against men, and an increase in what, in the past, would have been considered inappropriate sexual conduct, but is now defined as rape. These issues are discussed in more detail in the final chapter.

CHAPTER 2

Sexual Coercion, Sexual Assault, and Sexual Abuse

Sexual Coercion in Dating Relationships

"Boy, I've been watchin you like the hawk in the sky that fly/Boy you are my Prey" sings Aaliyah Timbaland in the hit song, "Are you that Somebody." In a Destiny's Child rap song called "Independent Women," the lyrics were equally aggressive: "Only ring you celly when I'm feelin lonely/When it's all over please get up and leave."

These songs were cited in a *New York Times* Sunday Times article, "She's Got to Be a Macho Girl,"[1] which was subtitled: "In a Role Reversal, Teenage Girls Are the Aggressors When It Comes to Boys."

One can cite hundreds of songs by male singers and songwriters that expressed the same kind of sentiment. The Rolling Stones' "Under My Thumb" comes to mind, but then, your author is from an earlier generational stock! From World War II comes "You Can't Say NO to a Soldier," with the encouragement to "heed the call to arms" and "You'd better give in if you want him to win for you." Joan Merrill sings the song in the 1942 movie musical, *Iceland*, in which a marine corporal is relentlessly pursued by a woman. Indeed, it would likely take a musicologist to innumerate all the examples of what might be called aggressive or even overly aggressive pursuit by women or men in song, and then even further back, there are examples from Shakespeare or Chaucer, as well as examples of bawdy limericks and poems that span human history. Indeed, whether it is a man or a woman depicted as "overly aggressive" in pursuit of sex is perhaps more a matter of style rather than substance, when it comes to popular cultural expression.

But, if the times are changing as they always have, are we truly experiencing something new in terms of dating, pursuit, and the relative aggressiveness of the sexes? Or, is it simply the current manifestation of a cultural shift that waxes and wanes in generational waves as to what are socially acceptable behavior and mores?

We perhaps need to be reminded that there was a time in the United States when very short skirts were the style; there was a "wild" new kind of music with accompanying new risqué dances; the political left was on the rise with a "police riot" against them in Chicago. There was widespread defiance of the law against a banned intoxicant; the women's movement demanded new rights, and young people had freedom to have sex without their parents knowing about it in a way that was simply not possible before, with less risk for pregnancy. We speak here about the 1920s and 1930s—not the 1960s and the early 1970s. The banned intoxicant was alcohol, not marijuana, condoms became more available, and in what some historians called a sea change of epic proportions—it was the advent of the car that got young people out from under the watchful eyes of parents where "spooning" was previously confined to the front porch or front parlor.

Even earlier, there was the socially acceptable practice of Bundling. Distances were large between courting couples. You could not send the suitor home after a "date" when they might live many days travel away. Incredible today, with the acquiescence of parents, an adolescent boy and girl were allowed to sleep together, usually at her parents' home. It originated apparently in the Netherlands and was practiced fairly commonly in colonial America, particularly in Pennsylvania. Sometimes, a bundling board was used, which was placed between them to prevent actual sexual intercourse—it was hoped.

It's Scary

As we have briefly explored, it is not that sexual pursuit by both sexes is substantially different today compared to previous generations. What is socially acceptable as a standard does seem to change. It was terrible behavior in some generations for a woman to "call" on a man first, even before the advent of the telephone. Apparently though, it was all right to drop her handkerchief for him to pick up and introduce himself.

In the *New York Times* article, the reporter interviewed a 16-year-old high school student by the name of John Bernard about the girls at his school: "They have more attitude. They have more power. And they overpower guys more. I mean, it's Scary." "*It's Scary*" is the operative phrase that we wish to explore here.

Sexual pursuit is one thing, and human beings seem to be limited in this pursuit only by the extent of their imagination. The use of coercion to obtain sexual desires is another matter. One would hope it is rarer. Coercion is scary.

What Is Coercion?

Coercion is defined by *West's Encyclopedia of American Law*[2] as "The intimidation of a victim to compel the individual to do some act against his or her will by the use of *psychological pressure* (emphasis added), physical force, or threats. The crime of intentionally and unlawfully restraining another's freedom by threatening to commit a crime, accusing the victim of a crime, disclosing any secret that would seriously impair the victim's reputation in the community. . . . A marriage may be annulled or a separation or divorce granted on the grounds of coercion."

Philosophers from the *Stanford Encyclopedia of Philosophy*, as we would expect, have a more expansive view of the term: "Sometimes the term 'coercion' is used in popular speech with a quite broad sense. For instance, one hears 'coercion' used to describe social pressures (e.g., the need to conform to peer expectations or to placate one's parents); or the constraining or manipulative effects of advertising, one's upbringing, or the structuring of society more generally (e.g., the necessity of participating in a capitalist economy). It is also sometimes treated as a quite general concept encompassing almost any sort of interpersonal infringement on one's rights."[3]

The *New World Encyclopedia*[4] defines it, in part, this way:

> In Aristotle's theory of moral responsibility there is no hard and fast rule for determining whether a person who has acted from coercion is blameworthy. It is important to notice that since coerced acts are always strictly voluntary, they are never automatically disqualified from responsibility. Responsibility depends on facts about the situation such as the gravity of the threat and the nature of the coerced act. For example, Aristotle holds it absurd that one could be coerced into killing one's mother.
>
> Most contemporary philosophers would agree with Aristotle. However, they have sought a specification of the conditions under which it does so. According to Harry Frankfurt, "a coercive threat arouses in its victim a desire—that is, to avoid the penalty—so powerful that it will move him to perform the required

action whether he wants to perform it or considers that it would be reasonable for him to do so." Most philosophers reject Frankfurt's analysis—at least as specifying a necessary condition for coercion—on the grounds that there are less extreme cases in which a person's will is hardly over-ridden, and yet she/he can be said to have been coerced. . . . In other words, Frankfurt's analysis picks out certain extreme cases, but fails to accommodate others. In particular, a person is coerced insofar as his will is overridden by a powerful desire arising from the coercive threat. However, many other theorists have insisted that this is incomplete: Features of the *environment* in which the agent acts are crucial in determining responsibility. Moreover, the strength of the threat, as well as severity of the consequences of non-compliance, in relation to the result (harm) of the demanded action must be weighed.[5]

Before we get too complicated, however, our first one-sentence legal definition would seem to suffice for most of the circumstances we are examining here: "The intimidation of a victim to compel the individual to do some act against his or her will by the use of psychological pressure, physical force, or threats." Blackmail, however, is often cited as an example of coercion, although it is generally prosecuted as a separate crime. Blackmail in the social sense, as in, "If you don't want to do it with me, then I'll tell everyone you are a wimp," certainly falls within our definition.

The National Intimate Partner and Sexual Violence Survey (NISVS) is a new (released in November 2011) large-scale nationally representative investigation into sexual coercion and other issues.

We will refer to this research extensively and repeat much of it verbatim due to it being a publically available government document (Centers for Disease Control and Prevention). It is unprecedented in a number of ways. The NISVS asked questions that had not been asked previously in such a large-scale survey. As importantly (and as we explored in the previous chapter on rape—at times inappropriately), it defined sexual coercion terms. We can expect that researchers will accede to these definitions due to the prestigious source and that such definitions will likely have an impact on the law:

- **Sexual coercion** is defined as unwanted sexual penetration that occurs after a person is pressured in a nonphysical way. In NISVS, sexual coercion refers to unwanted vaginal, oral, or anal sex after being pressured in ways that included being worn down by someone who repeatedly asked for sex or showed they were unhappy; feeling pressured by being lied to, being told promises that were untrue, having someone threaten to end a relationship or spread rumors; and sexual pressure due to someone using their influence or authority.

- **Unwanted sexual contact** is defined as unwanted sexual experiences involving touch but not sexual penetration, such as being kissed in a sexual way, or having sexual body parts fondled or grabbed.
- **Non-contact unwanted sexual experiences** are those unwanted experiences that do not involve any touching or penetration, including someone exposing their sexual body parts, flashing, or masturbating in front of the victim, someone making a victim show his or her body parts, someone making a victim look at or participate in sexual photos or movies, or someone harassing the victim in a public place in a way that made the victim feel unsafe.[6]

A Shift in Young Attitudes?

Also quoted in the previously discussed *New York Times* article is Dr. Ann Kearney-Cooke. She is the co-director of the Helping Girls Become Strong Women Project at Columbia University. She maintains that things are different now for teenage girls because of societal shifts: "The culture—MTV videos and television shows—helps to reduce adolescent girls to being successful when they look sexy and date often. There is a status to the girl in middle school who is the first one to start dating. One of the ways we learn about relationships is by being in them and seeing them. Today, kids come home from school and the parents or parent might not be home. They watch MTV and talk shows and cruise the internet, and that is where they are learning about relationships." As paraphrased by the reporter, Kearney-Cooke was inclined to believe that, "Girls are indeed becoming sexually and romantically more aggressive for several reasons, including the unintended consequences of their equal upbringing." She pointed out that girls are becoming more like boys and that several studies show they now equal them in smoking and drinking.[7]

Using the 2005 Youth Risk Behavior Survey (YRBS), funded by the CDC, 10.8 percent of girls and 4.2 percent of boys report that they were forced to have sexual intercourse when they did not want to.[8]

The 2004 Boston Youth Survey (BYS) survey documents the aggressive behavior by both boys and girls in the Boston school system.[9] The survey is the result of a collaborative effort between the Harvard Youth Violence Prevention Center and the Boston Office of Human Services and Boston Youth & Families. The Sexual Abuse and Dating Violence section of the BYS survey paints a dramatically different picture than the one presented (passive females and aggressive males) by most domestic violence organizations. The BYS notes that 7 percent of girls and 5 percent of boys over their lifetime report experiencing sexual violence by their dating partner.

In fact, the BYS data is consistent with national data that has been available for years from the national YRBS (Centers for Disease Control and Prevention, 2006).[10] The YRBS documents that 10.8 percent of girls and 4.2 percent of teenage boys were physically forced to have sexual intercourse against their will with a dating partner.

Aggression

A comparison of men and women's aggression in general, and in particular within intimate partner relationships, was discussed in great detail in, *Abused Men: The Hidden Side of Domestic Violence*. It is sufficient here to say that it is richly referenced and the case is proven that there is gender symmetry when it comes to intimate partner violence, be it young dating couples or those married or cohabitating. The question of whether women in general are becoming *more* aggressive than they have in the past, which may lead to criminal or detrimental behavior to themselves or others, also is proven. For example, for the first time since the U.S. Justice Department began keeping records, women now surpass men for convictions in one criminal activity—embezzlement. And as discussed in the previous volume, researchers predict that women will eventually equal men in all crime areas except for stranger-to-stranger homicide. Details on this result and a discussion of aggression in general and in intimate partner relationships may be found in *Abused Men: The Hidden Side of Domestic Violence*.

Measuring whether or not women's sexual aggression is *increasing* in recent years, particularly in dating relationships must, unfortunately, be generally relegated to anecdotal accounts of men and perceptions of teachers and professors such as Kearney-Cooke. In other words, we do not have a strong basis over a significant period of time. The study of sexual behavior involving coercion and assault in dating relationships is relatively new, particularly in regards to male victimization, so we do not have available truly long-term comparisons.

Dating Coercion Research

However, thanks to the work of one researcher, we do have a good picture of what the research has unearthed thus far. This does not include the previously mentioned Centers for Disease Control and Prevention's NISVS because it is so new. It is important, however, to examine as much research as possible that was developed prior to the CDC report. Martin Fiebert PhD/MFCC is a Clinical Psychologist at California State University, Long Beach. Dr. Fiebert completed his undergraduate work at Queens College, New York in 1960 and received his doctorate from the University of Rochester, New York in 1965. Since then, he has been a professor at Cal State Long Beach, California as well as the president of the Long Beach Chapter of the California Faculty Association (CFA) during 2001–2003. One of his areas of specialty is Gender Studies: Psychology of Male Roles. Dr. Fiebert has written numerous scholarly articles. In 2003 and 2004, he was selected as an International Scientist of the Year. He is perhaps best known for his extraordinary work in developing and maintaining the references examining *Assaults by Women on Their Spouses or Male Partners: An Annotated Bibliography*,[11] which demonstrates that women are as physically aggressive, or more aggressive, than men in their relationships with their spouses or male partners. This bibliography examines 282 scholarly investigations—218 empirical studies and 64 reviews and/or analyses. The aggregate sample size in the reviewed studies exceeds 369,800.

Not as nearly well-known is a similar annotated bibliography by Fiebert titled *References Examining Men as Victims of Women's Sexual Coercion*.[12] Forty empirical studies and two reviews listed demonstrate that men also experience sexual coercion. Fiebert's important and essential work can be examined via the link noted in note (12) referenced above. As new research becomes available, readers can rely on updates.

Despite these studies, what we know is still limited. Almost all of the research involves college-age students. Although, as noted earlier, there are good data on middle and high school students available, such as the YRBS. It is, however, a lot easier to measure the college student population. The students fill out the survey because it is part of a class assignment or there may be small fee incentives for participation and student helpers such as graduate students are available to collate the results. Despite the general limitations due to this population, it is instructive to examine some typical results.

One example is a survey from the University of Washington by the Addictive Behaviors Research Center and reported in the journal *Sex*

Roles, but after the college produced a news release, the report also reached a far wider audience as it was reported in detail in the *Seattle Post Intelligencer*, a daily newspaper at the time.[13] They asked questions of just a subset of the college population—fraternity and sorority pledges. We assume the researchers chose this particular group because of the assumption that these students are perhaps known to participate in particularly wild parties where alcohol is consumed and sexual advances are also likely to take place.

Male students reported "unwanted" sexual contact and coercion in rates similar to that of women. The questionnaire measured five types—from feeling pressured to have sex to physical force. Twenty-one percent of the men and 28 percent of the women said they had experienced at least one of the five types. Men were more likely to use force, drugs, or alcohol to get sex, but were also more likely to feel pressured to have sex when they did not want to. Less than 1 percent of the men reported physical force while 5 percent of the women did, defined as someone "twisting your arm or holding you down."

The full results are shown in Table 2.1.

Mary Larimer was an assistant professor of psychology and principal investigator at the time of survey. She told the newspaper, " Initially, it was surprising to me." In a news release, she said, "Both men and women are experiencing unwanted sexual advances, and our preliminary indications are that men are suffering from these experiences just as much as women. I was surprised at how guilty and ashamed some of the men were and that we, as researchers, were buying into a cultural myth and didn't think such experiences were the same for men as for women."

Table 2.1   Unwanted Sex (NISVS)

	Men	Women
Unwanted sexual contact	21%	28%
Unwanted sex because partner was aroused	14%	8%
Pressured into unwanted sex by continual arguments	8%	6%
Partner attempted intercourse using physical force	<1%	5%
Partner attempted intercourse after giving drugs/alcohol	9%	17%
Unwanted sex after being given drugs/alcohol	4%	6%
Alcohol led to sexual situation later regretted	47%	48%

Other studies from the Fiebert bibliography and other sources paint a similar picture. We can break the results down in areas of particular interest, as discussed in the following sections.

Largest Sample Size

The most common size of the sampled college students were in the 300–400 participant range. The apparent largest was reported in *The Psychological of Women Quarterly*,[14] with data collected from 1,192 men and 2,742 women at a large midwestern university. In addition to undergraduates, graduates, faculty, and staff were included. The results indicate that 49 percent of women and 24 percent of men had experienced at least one unwanted sexual behavior, although the sample size included twice as many women.

Typical Results

In the *Journal of Family Issues*,[15] we find that in a response to a nine-question survey, the undergraduates revealed that 38 percent of men and 30 percent of women experienced at least one instance of sexual coercion in the previous 12-month period. Of particular interest in this study, questions were also asked about perpetrator behavior. Men said they were the aggressor to a greater extent than women did, 37 percent versus 18 percent of the women.

In the *Journal of College Student Development*,[16] responses to a "Sexual Experience Survey" found that 15 percent of men and 25 percent of women had engaged in sexual intercourse at least once "when they did not want to because of psychological or verbal coercion."

This is, of course, behavior that is not the same as rape. Such results, particularly of the latter type, have been frequently used by some advocates to claim that one in four women or one in five have been raped while on campus. Using the same data, a different kind of advocate could claim it is one in seven or eight male rape victims. We will discuss this issue in further detail in our final chapter.

In *Violence and Victims*,[17] the students completed a survey examining unwanted sexual behavior as a function of 12 coercive techniques including intoxication, false promises, threats, and physical force. Men reported 457 incidents and women reported 628. The most common techniques experienced by both genders were intoxication and persistent touching. Men were more likely than women to experience unwanted sexual behavior when their partners used blackmail. In general, however, women were coerced into more extreme sexual behaviors than men. The American College Health Association report, *Campus Violence White Paper*, documents that 15 percent of females and 9.2 percent of males report being in an emotionally abusive relationship. Also, 2.4 percent of females and 1.3 percent of males have been in a physically abusive relationship and 1.7 percent of females and 1 percent of males have been in a sexually abusive relationship within the last school year.[18]

Other Countries

There are not very many comparisons between other countries and U.S. college students in this regard. A direct comparison was made in the *Journal of Sex Research*[19] between Swedish and U.S. students. The results were that 50 percent of the U.S. men compared to 22 percent of the Swedish men and 69 percent of the U.S. women compared to 41 percent of the Swedish women reported that they were subjected to at least one sexually coercive strategy in the previous 12 months.

Race

Some researchers have examined whether there are differences between various ethnic groups regarding sexually coercive behavior. In the *Journal of Adolescent Health*,[20] a survey among a younger group (middle and high school students) was conducted. They found that 18 percent of females and 12 percent of males reported having an unwanted sexual experience, and that among the ethnic groups, Asians (7%) reported having had such an incident less frequently than non-Hispanic white (16%), Hispanic (16%), or black (19%) students. The researchers, while examining race, did not include details on gender.

In the *Journal of College Student Development*,[21] men were significantly more likely than women to report that their partner "pressured them for sex," and "got angry if refused." However, this gender difference was present only for whites and blacks, but not for Hispanics.

Response and Perceptions

A number of researchers have examined how female and male students respond to or perceive sexually coercive actions. Most typically, this is done with having the students view drawings, videos, or descriptions (vignettes) in which situations were presented and then gauging the reaction. In the journal *Sex Roles*,[22] six vignettes were presented in which both genders were depicted as aggressors and victims. Male participants saw the sexual advances as more coercive when the victim was female, while females saw the advances as more coercive when the victim was male.

In the *Archives of Sexual Behavior*,[23] in an article titled "Gender and the Stolen Kiss," a vignette was presented in which one dating partner indicates that he/she does not want to be kissed and the other partner does not listen. There was significantly more support for women to violate men's sexual consent and less support for men than women to withhold sexual consent to be kissed. The *Journal of Sex Research*[24] reports that the main reasons men engaged in unwanted sexual behavior compared to women were peer pressure and the desire for popularity. Interestingly, this survey reported the highest totals of both men and women reporting having engaged in unwanted sexual intercourse, with significantly more men (63%) than women (46%) reporting this, and even higher totals reporting some form of unwanted sexual activity (97% women, 93% men).

In another paper in the *Journal of Sex Research*,[25] the findings indicate that male victims of female sexual assaults were judged more likely to have encouraged the sexual acts, were assumed to have enjoyed it more, and believed to be less stressed than female victims.

In the journal *Sex Roles*,[26] 300 male and female college students were presented with a vignette in which they imagined an uninvited genital touch, either gentle or forceful, from either a male or female college acquaintance. Findings revealed that women anticipated strong negative effects from receiving such a touch, whether gentle or forceful, while men anticipated little negative effect from either kind of touch. Both genders responded negatively to opposite gender touching. The same study was used to examine only male reactions involving a moderately forceful sexual advance from a female casual acquaintance. The men's sexual standards, relationship availability, and the attractiveness of the sexual initiator were studied. More positive responses were obtained from men with less restrictive sexual standards, who had no girlfriend, and who were told that the female initiator was attractive. The majority of men, however, reacted negatively to the coercive situation.

As acknowledged by Dr. Malcolm George in his paper for this volume and by others, researcher Cindy Struckman-Johnson at the University of South Dakota and David Struckman-Johnson have been pioneers in asking questions of men as well as women. While the subject has been studied from the 1950s to the 1980s, it was only in the context of female victims and male perpetrators—it was not until the late 1980s that the same types of questions were also asked of males.

In a 2003 paper for the Society for the Scientific Study of Sexuality, the Struckman-Johnsons presented their findings from a recent survey of college students at a Midwestern and a Southern university. Their conclusions about their research, and just as importantly, the demonstration in their paper that their results are consistent with other surveys of college students, found that

> Most frequently reported tactics across genders. Although there were fewer perpetrators than receivers, the two groups showed similar patterns for the most frequently occurring tactics. . . . There were no gender differences for sexual outcome of the most recent incident among the receivers or among the perpetrators. The most recent incident resulted in sexual intercourse for 48% of receivers and 55% of perpetrators.[27]

In other words, *a substantial number (48%) of the students engaged in sexual intercourse even though they had raised objections to coercive tactics.* Real descriptions of what happens on campus are rare in the academic literature, but this paper does include a good sample. Here are some selected highlights:

> We had "made out" the weekend before, but I didn't want to continue any further . . . She got drunk and so did I. . . . She wanted to "hook up again." But I thought it was a bad idea. She pinned me down at one point . . . but I left.

> I told her no and she kept kissing me and touching me. She kept asking and trying to make me have sex with her. I was drunk and tried to leave. She stood in front of the door, she slapped me and let me go calling me names as I walked away.

> I locked the room door that we were in. I kissed and touched him. I removed his shirt and unzipped his pants. He asked me to stop. I didn't. Then, I sat on top of him. He had had two beers but wasn't drunk.

> It was like this: She, before engaging in sex, asked me if it wasn't just a one-night stand. I told her no, it wasn't. At the time I thought I meant it. . . . Maybe the liquor?

We were at her parents' house getting intoxicated. She went to "go take a shower," but came out of the bathroom with only a robe on. She removed it and was naked and tried to grope me.

She asked me to bring her to the bank to get some money which was close to my house. We went to my apartment where she tried to kiss me. I told her to quit. She then grabbed my genitals and I quickly removed her hand. She then took off her clothes and said take me. I laughed at her. She asked why didn't I want her. I replied because I have a girlfriend. Then she kept pushing the issue until I gave in.

Beyond College

As we have determined, finding research that goes beyond surveying what college students report in terms of sexual coercion is much rarer. Apparently, the first and one of the few surveys of adult employed women and their attitudes towards coercive sexual tactics was developed by the researchers at the University of Guelph in the *Journal of Sex Research* and reported to a wider public in the Canadian newspaper, the *National Post*.[28]

Psychology professor Serge Desmarais told the paper, "Women are sexual beings, though there seems to be an effort, somewhere, to avoid talking about that topic." Desmarais told the reporter he is about as "pro-feminist as you can get." He contended that because women resort to sexual pressure tactics, it does not change the fact that "male coercion has far more impact and is felt with tremendous pain in women's lives." Fellow researcher Michele Clements-Schreiber said that dismissing men's experiences or regarding coercion as normal carries with it a danger to women: "Trivializing men's experiences may invite men also to dismiss women's non-violent coercive experiences." Clements-Schreiber says her interest in research into this area began when she was talking to her two teenage boys about dating behavior and she heard this response from one of her sons, " 'You're always telling me all of these things, but why is that everyone seems to think it's OK for a woman to do whatever she wants' And I said to him, 'No of course that's not OK. Pressure is pressure, whether it comes from a woman or a man." Clements-Schreiber also told the reporter, "To fail to recognize that women are willing to use some pressure to get a sexually reluctant partner is to infer that sex is one of those things that women just don't want. And I don't buy that."

The results of the survey are instructive, the women were asked if they have ever used certain pressure tactics with a reluctant or unwilling male partner, as well as about their attitudes toward using such tactics:

Begin to undress him—48%
Undo his shirt and kiss or nibble on his chest—58%
Undo his belt or pants—51%
Push him onto the bed and begin to undress him—40%
Get him a little bit drunk—26%
It is more difficult for men to tell the difference between love and lust—46%
Women should be able to have sex when they want it—47%
The truth is that men enjoy getting sexual advances from women, even when they do not respond positively—65%

The Centers for Disease Control and Prevention NISVS Results on Coercion

About 1 in 8 women (13%) reported experiencing sexual coercion in her lifetime, which translates to more than 15 million women in the United States. Sexual coercion was reported by 2.0% of women in the 12 months prior to taking the survey, six percent of men (almost 7 million men), and 1.5% in the 12 months prior to taking the survey.

Unwanted Sexual Contact

More than one-quarter of women (27.2%) have experienced some form of unwanted sexual contact in their lifetime. This equates to over 32 million women in the United States. The 12 month prevalence of unwanted sexual contact reported by women was 2.2%. *Approximately 1 in 9 men (11.7%) reported experiencing unwanted sexual contact in his lifetime, which translates to an estimated 13 million men in the United States* (emphasis added). The 12 month prevalence of unwanted sexual contact reported by men was 2.3%.

Sexual Experiences

Non-contact unwanted sexual experiences were the most common form of sexual violence experienced by both women and men. One-third of women (33.7%) experienced some type of noncontact unwanted sexual experience in their lifetime, and 1 in 33 women (3.0%) experienced this in the 12 months prior to taking the survey. This equates to 40 million women in the United States for the lifetime estimate and 3.5 million women in the last 12 months. Nearly 1 in 8 men (12.8%) reported non-contact unwanted sexual experiences in his lifetime, and 1 in 37 men (2.7%) experienced this type of sexual violence in the 12 months before taking the survey. *These numbers translate to 14 million men in the United States who have had these experiences in their lifetime and 3 million men in the last 12 months* (emphasis added).

The gender discrepancies in "lifetime experiences" versus the near equanimity in the genders "during the last 12 months," suggest the possibility either that females have increased their involvement in these activities in the last few years or males have decreased their involvement.

Sexual Violence Other than Rape—According to the CDC National Intimate Partner and Sexual Violence Survey

For both women and men, the type of perpetrator varied by the form of sexual violence experienced. The majority of female victims of sexual coercion and unwanted sexual contact reported known perpetrators. Three-quarters of female victims (75.4%) of sexual coercion reported perpetration by an intimate partner, and nearly 1 in 2 female victims (45.9%) of unwanted sexual contact reported perpetration by an acquaintance. Strangers were the most commonly reported perpetrators of non-contact unwanted sexual experiences against women, reported by 1 in 2 female victims (50.5%).

Male victims most commonly reported a known perpetrator for all types of sexual violence other than rape. Nearly half of male victims reported an intimate partner (44.8%) or an acquaintance (44.7%) as a perpetrator in situations where the male was made to penetrate someone else. The majority of male victims of sexual coercion (69.7%) reported an intimate partner as a perpetrator. For both unwanted sexual contact (51.7%) and non-contact unwanted sexual experiences (44.9%), approximately 1 in 2 male victims reported an acquaintance as a perpetrator.

A majority of male victims reported only female perpetrators (emphasis added): being made to penetrate (79.2%), sexual coercion (83.6%), and unwanted sexual contact (53.1%). For non-contact unwanted sexual experiences, approximately half of male victims (49.0%) reported only male perpetrators and more than one-third (37.7%) reported only female perpetrators.[29]

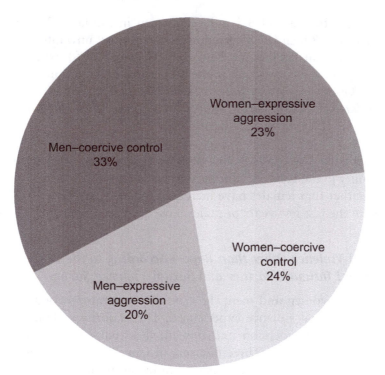

Graph 2.1   NISVS 2010 Victims of Psychological Aggression

Further analysis of the CDC survey is provided by Bert Hoff of the University of Phoenix (Graph 2.1):

Men were more often the victims of both psychological aggression ("expressive aggression" and "coercive control") and control of reproductive or sexual health. Name-calling is one of the forms of "expressive aggression," which included acting angry in a way that seemed dangerous, name-calling and insulting remarks. The other category of "psychological aggression" is "coercive control," such as restricting access to friends or relatives and having to account for all of one's time. *In the last 12 months, 20,548,000 men (18.1%) and 16,578,000 (13.9%) women were subjected to psychological aggression* (emphasis added). For women, this was split fairly evenly between expressive aggression and coercive control, while for men, 15.2% were subjected to coercive control and 9.3% to expressive aggression. The main forms of expressive aggression against women were insults (64.3%) and name-calling (58.0%). For men the top items were being called names (51.6%) and being told they were losers (42.4%).[30]

Whether or not such actions should be labeled "violence" was the subject debated with the CDC in the previous chapter. We now turn our attention to types of assaults that can be more accurately called violence.

Sexual Assault and Abuse

Jim screamed in pain. He and his wife had just finished having sexual intercourse and she was on top of him. When she got off of him, she took her long fingernails and deeply scratched his penis, leaving bloody marks and wounds. After the attack, she laughed.

They eventually divorced, and the sexual assault was simply part of a long history of various types of physical abuse. Jim, an emergency medicine technician, never told anyone about what had happened to him, and treated himself for the injuries.

Tom, was married for 13 years, and suffered many types of physical abuse from his wife. Most of this involved her throwing things as well as verbal put-downs. She also sexually abused him. She kicked him in the testicles at least once that he can recall, and then used her long fingernails to dig deeply into his arm and shoulder, insisting that he join her and another couple in having sex. This was something he did not want to do, but he complied.

Almost everyone has heard the story of Lorena Bobbitt. In June of 1993, John Wayne Bobbitt was intoxicated when he came home to the couple's apartment in Virginia. According to court testimony given by Lorena Bobbitt, he raped her. In a 1994 trial, though, he was found innocent of the alleged rape. Just after the alleged rape, and according to her account, she grabbed a kitchen knife and while he was sleeping, cut off almost half of his penis. After the assault, she left the apartment with the severed penis and threw it into a field. It was only after this that she stopped the car she was driving and called 911. The police searched the field, found the penis and packed it in ice. It took a nine-hour operation to reattach the penis.

The media attention the case attracted, the nightly jokes on the *Tonight Show* and other outlets, is a matter of record.

It is worthwhile here, however, to note that while the Bobbitt case received the most media attention at the time, there have been other similar cases. In 2011, for example, we found three other cases of sexual assault involving penis removal:

- In January of that year, Liu Nuo of Xi'an, China, cut off the penis of her husband Dong Feng with a knife. She was arrested.
- In February, Chen Jian of Sydney, Australia, allegedly served sleeping drug–laced soup to her former boyfriend, Xian Peng. When he fell asleep, she allegedly tied his hands and feet, sliced his penis off, and stabbed him. He later died. She faces murder charges in Australia.

Deserving of special attention due to it occurring in the United States and the attendant media attention and reaction it received, is the criminal case of Catherine Kieu Becker of Garden Grove, California. According to *Los Angeles Times* reports, on July 4, she cut off her husband's penis with a 10-inch kitchen knife. Following the pattern of other female penis cutters, her methodology included drugging her husband's dinner to make him sleepy and then tying him to the bed. When he awoke, she cut off his penis, tossed it in the garbage disposal and turned it on. Garden Grove police Lt. Jeff Nightengale said, "He was conscious when his penis was removed." He said Kieu called police to report a medical emergency and told arriving officers, "he deserved it," before pointing to the room where the victim was found bleeding profusely. The 60-year-old man had filed for divorce from his wife in May, but they were still living together at the time of the assault. District Attorney chief of staff, Susan King said, "It's hard to believe what would motivate a person to do this sort of thing. It's one of the worst things you could do to a person short of killing him." Police did not reveal the victim's name and he was taken to a local hospital where surgery was performed. Citing patient privacy, the hospital has not revealed whether the penis was reattached, but given the fact that it was tossed in a garbage disposal, it seems unlikely. Catherine Kieu was charged with torture and aggravated mayhem. She could face life in prison without the possibility of parole.[31]

The *Washington Post* described the reaction of television talk show panelists to this crime not long after it occurred. On the national CBS television show, *The Talk*: "I don't know the circumstances," host Sharon Osbourne said. "However, I do think it's quite fabulous." What sounded like the entire audience began to laugh. The other panelists— Leah Remini, Julie Chen, Holly Robinson Peete, and Sara Gilbert—did not revel in the story quite as much. But all of the hosts let out at least a small chuckle during the conversation.

Gilbert pointed out that the conversation could be perceived as sexist. "Not to be a total buzz kill," Gilbert began, "but it is a little bit sexist. If somebody cut a woman's breast off, nobody would be sitting laughing." "It's different," Osbourne said, before comparing the two parts of the anatomy.[32] On July 19, Osbourne discussed her behavior, stating *between spurts of laughter* that she was "sorry that she offended people" and that she did "not condone genital mutilation."[33]

As we can see by these incidents, sexual assault by women against men covers a wide range. It is not just limited to the more sensational type of penis-cutting assault, though certainly, these types of rare incidents are more likely to garner news media attention precisely because they do not happen very often. However, the more common type of sexual assault against men (kicking or hitting his testicles, threatening to kick or hit or having objects thrown at his groin area—often with an accompanying laugh track) is an almost nightly affair on many types of television shows.

What Are Sexual Assault and Sexual Abuse?

It is notable that this type of sexual assault in which men are kicked or hit in the groin area is not considered sexual assault by many researchers. It is the question *not* asked. Often, it is not even classified as a physical assault.

A good example of this is the National Violence Against Women Survey, which was funded by the U.S. Justice Department and the CDC. This survey is one of the largest of its kind and is often used as a source for citing the extent and nature of rape, sexual assault, and intimate partner violence.[34] As noted in a previous work, *Abused Men: The Hidden Side of Domestic Violence,* 36 percent of the respondents who were victims of severe intimate partner violence were men.

For our purposes here, however, it is notable that the questions about assault put to both men and women did not include questions about some of the common assaults that men face, particularly by intimate partners. That is, having boiling or hot liquids (being "intentionally burned"—not defined further—was used as a type of intimate partner violence attack in the new CDC National Intimate Partner and Sexual Violence Survey) used against them, being scratched, poisoning or attempted poisoning, soliciting or using another person to carry out an attack, and being kicked or punched in the groin or having objects thrown at the groin area. In other words, if the question is never asked, then the phenomenon does not exist. The question of *why* these researchers, prosecutors, and others fail to include groin attacks against males as a type of sexual assault cannot be readily answered. Making an assumption about motives is a dangerous game, but it may fall into the category of intentional or unintentional neglect.

A central problem also, is that most research mixes child sexual abuse with adult-to-adult sexual abuse. Therefore, it can be extremely difficult to isolate the two from each other.

For example, L. A. Johnson in a doctoral dissertation defined covert and overt sexual abuse:

- Covert abuse includes age-inappropriate bathing, cleaning excessively, bathing together, wiping, enemas, sleeping with the intent of intimacy, French kissing, seductive behaviors, sensual massages, spanking for pleasure, excessive holding, kissing, caressing, voyeurism, forcing to watch pornography, or making pornography.
- Overt abuse includes digital–genital contact with or without penetration, oral–genital contact, insertion of objects, masturbating in front of the person, forcing them to watch sexual activities, forcing them to engage in sexual activities with others.[35]

Obviously, sexual abuse can only be defined as such in what Johnson calls the "covert" arena when it is perpetrated against children, but would not be considered as sexual abuse between adults, except perhaps in terms of being forced to watch pornography or taking pornographic pictures without consent.

Canadian law defines sexual assault in a number of ways:

"Somebody touches you in a sexual way *on purpose,* directly or indirectly, *without your consent.* . . . Somebody sexually assaults you and is armed with, or uses, a weapon, or, forces you to have sex by threatening to do injury to somebody else, (for example: they threaten to hurt your brother or sister if you don't do it), or, they injure you. . . . Aggravated Sexual Assault—Somebody sexually assaults you and they cause serious injuries to you." Interestingly, Canadian law adds this statement: "You can't legally consent to have sex with someone who is in a position of trust, power or authority over you, for example, a minister, coach, employer, teacher, police officer."[36]

It is worthwhile here, to examine that last statement and compare it to commonplace situations. Does this mean that consent is always absent when a boss marries or has sex with a subordinate? Can police officers only marry other police officers and only if they are of the same rank? If the religion is not Catholicism, can ministers not have sex with or marry a parishioner? It may be in many cases that it is against university policy for college teachers to have a sexual relationship with a college student (particularly if the teacher is grading that student). However, to believe that this is an uncommon occurrence or believe that the adult student can never truly consent to a sexual relationship or cohabit with or marry a teacher is absurd. If one cannot "legally consent" to have sex with anyone who has a "position of trust, power and authority over you," certainly prohibits a lot of fairly common romantic relationships.

In the United States, the legal definition of sexual assault varies from state to state. The Rape, Abuse & Incest National Network defines sexual assault as "unwanted sexual contact that stops short of rape or attempted rape. This includes sexual touching and fondling."[37]

The National Center for Victims of Crime says it is: "Any Unwanted sexual contact or threats. Usually a sexual assault occurs when someone touches any part of another person's body in a sexual way, even through clothes, without that person's consent."[38]

The U.S. Federal Criminal Code[39] defines two kinds of sexual assault, Abuse and Aggravated sexual abuse.

Sexual abuse is defined by action that causes another person to "Engage in a sexual activity by threatening or placing that person in fear. Engaging in a sexual act if that person is incapable of declining participation in, or communicating unwillingness to engage in that sexual act."

There is a further definition of what is called Abusive Sexual Contact: "When no sexual penetration actually occurred but when the intentional touching. . . of the genitalia, anus, groin, breast, inner thigh, or buttocks of any person with an intent to abuse, humiliate, harass, degrade, or arouse or gratify the sexual desire of any person occurs." Aggravated Sexual Abuse is defined as: "When a person knowingly causes another person to engage in a sexual act. . . or attempts to do so by using force against that person, or by threatening or placing that person in fear that that person will be subjected to death, serious bodily injury, or kidnapping." The Federal Code also defines what is meant by Aggravated Sexual Abuse by Other Means: "When a person knowingly renders another person unconscious and thereby engages in a sexual act with that other person; or administers to another person by force or threat of force, or without the knowledge or permission of that person, a drug, intoxicant, or other similar substance and thereby: a) Substantially impairs the ability of that person to appraise or control conduct."

The Ridiculous Gets Serious

The Headline: School Backs Off Claim that Playground Touching by 6-Year-Old Was Sexual Assault

In California, a six-year-old boy was suspended for sexual assault after touching another boy during recess. "Levina Subrata spoke to the *New York Times* about the incident at Lupine Hills Elementary in Hercules, Calif. The school claimed Subrata's son had touched another boy on the thigh or groin; Subrata said the conduct was innocent. 'They were playing tag,' she told the *Times*. 'There's no intent to do any sort of sexual assault.'"

Eventually, the school did remove the sexual assault note from the boy's record, but only after the parents hired an attorney. "Experts told the *Times that such incidents are part of an emerging national trend* (emphasis added)."[40]

The Headline: First-Grader Suspended for Sexual Harassment

In Brockton, Massachusetts the first-grader was suspended for touching another first-grader underneath the waistband of her pants. His mother, Berthena Dorinvil, said he was too young to even understand what sexual harassment is: "What are you talking about? He's 6 years old," Dorinvil said. "I feel terrible. He feels terrible. He keeps telling me 'Mommy, are the police going to arrest me?' He's very emotional." The boy was suspended for three days. Brockton Superintendent of Schools Basan Nemirkow said, that the district takes all allegations of sexual harassment very seriously. Dorinvil said, "The girl said my son touched her waistband. That's what the girl said to the principal. My son said, no, he touched her back, just on her shirt, because the girl touched him first. . . . He was crying and said, 'Mommy, why is this a big deal? What is this? I thought we were all sisters and brothers in class.' "[41]

The Headline: Prosecutor of Bottom-Swatting Boys Is Arrested in Alleged Assault

In McMinnville, Oregon a bizarre series of events has ended with charges being brought against a county prosecutor who previously prosecuted two seventh-grade boys for swatting bottoms of girls at a middle school. Prosecutor Debra Markham was arrested in November of 2007, after allegedly punching her husband in the face. As a result of that incident, she is no longer a prosecutor. In the Summer of 2007, Markham had made national headlines with her prosecution of the boys. In response to news stories, people from around the nation sent the boys families more than $60,000 for a defense fund. A month after the case was filed, a judge dismissed the charges when a confidential out-of-court settlement was reached. The two boys spent five days in jail and were charged with felony sex abuse. They were expelled from school and could have faced up to ten years in juvenile jail and would have been placed on a sex offender registry for life. "Juvenile court records in the case showed both boys and girls were slapping one another's bottoms, and two of the girls identified as victims said they felt pressured by investigators to give false statements. . . .'I feel like karma has finally come back to Debra Markham for prosecuting Cory and Ryan,' said Tracie Mashburn, the mother of one of the boys."[42]

We will discuss in some detail the new (2011) U.S. Department of Education directive for colleges regarding procedures for sexual assault investigations in our final chapter. This is because the new directive has more to do with policy changes than incident accounts or data.

Suffice it to say, however, that the above three headline stories, as the *New York Times* article suggests, are part of a national trend and effects policy at all educational levels. We sourced the newspaper article from *The American Bar Association Journal* due to the fact that it was of enough interest to attorneys for it to be posted there, and because of the number of interesting comments it received—primarily, of course, from attorneys. Most of the comments were related to the idea that school districts have to investigate all such allegations as a defensive legal step.

One commentator signed themselves as "Attorney For a Board." "We actually had a lady come into our district and tell the principal at the school that she sued the last Board where her child was a student and she would sue ours. She did just that and while we prevailed it was still expensive to defend. Additionally, while the parents that sued may get taxed with costs, you generally never are able to recover them and attempting to do so is just more costly . . . While it does keep me in a paycheck, it can also get terribly annoying having to fight cases that you believe under the law should never have been filed . . . it becomes more cost efficient for the School Board to settle cases that they could win in court rather than litigating them to conclusion."[43]

The trivialization of sexual coercion, sexual assault, and sexual harassment incidents, as we will discuss throughout this volume, is not limited to the very young. Certainly, as the attorneys suggest, it can be traced to a more litigious climate in general and defensive legal maneuvers that do keep all attorneys in business. The climactic change, however, can also be attributed to a championed cause that has redefined male–female relations.

Consider, for example, these two questions from the National Intimate Partner and Sexual Violence Survey:

How many people have you had vaginal, oral or anal sex with after they pressured you by:

- Doing things like telling you lies, *making promises about the future they knew were untrue*, threatening to end your relationship, or threatening to spread rumors about you?
- Wearing you down by repeatedly asking for sex, or *showing they were unhappy*?[44]

The reader might pause for a moment here and think about their own experiences regarding their intimate relationships, and consider how they would answer these questions.

The CDC has a few more in this regard:

How many of your romantic or sexual partners have ever . . .

- Told you that you were a loser, a failure, or not good enough?
- Called you names like ugly, fat, crazy, or stupid?
- Insulted, humiliated, or made fun of you in front of others?
- Told you that no one else would want you?[45]

There were also a few other questions in this subject area—*exposed their sexual body parts, flashed you, masturbation in front of, making the other person show sexual body parts, and making someone else look at or participate in sexual photos or movies*. For some of these questions, the CDC interviewers put in "Remember, we are only asking about things that you didn't want to happen."

That caution, however, was not put in with every single question. The caution was usually grouped in a series of questions.

Saving the reader from having to go back and look at the total survey results by percentage, it is interesting to note here the representative sample survey results for the total U.S. population. Most importantly, note how the CDC defined the issue: Sexual *Violence* (emphasis added) Other Than Rape. They found a lifetime rate of *53 million women* and *25 million men*.

For sexual coercion, the total was 15 million women and 6 million men. For unwanted sexual contact, 32 million women–13 million men. For noncontact unwanted sexual experiences, it was 40 million women and 14 million men.

For the previous 12-month period, the results were:

	Women	Men
Sexual Coercion	*2.4 million*	*1.7 million*
Unwanted Sexual Contact	*2.6 million*	*2.6 million*
NonContact Unwanted Sexual Experience	*3.5 million*	*3.0 million*

Or, to put all this in another way:

"Nearly 1 in 2 women and 1 in 5 men experienced sexual violence victimization other than rape at some point in their lives." And "Approximately 1 in 20 women *and* (emphasis added) men experienced sexual violence victimization other than rape in the 12 months prior to taking the survey."[46]

Let us translate all this into what you will begin to see on the internet and even in what is called the mainstream news media. Certainly, these and similar statements will appear on advocacy groups websites and blogs:

Half of all women (50%) have experienced sexual violence!—Centers for Disease Control and Prevention

6.6 million women a year are sexually violated!—Centers for Disease Control and Prevention

One can also rightly assume that there will be no or little mention of the same survey results for males. After all, there are seven commissions for women in the federal government and none for men, most states have commissions for women (there is one state—New Hampshire—with a commission for men), including commissions on women's health, but none for men's health. The number of advocacy groups for women's concerns of all stripes are legion, while the number of such groups for men pale in comparison and they also receive considerably less financial support.

Coincidentally, there are also 7 million people in the United States who are currently under some form of correctional supervision, either imprisoned, on probation or parole.[47] Or, the number of women experiencing "sexual violence" each year is only slightly less than the number of criminals.

Are we not all of us now criminals?

Consider this again:

How many of your romantic or sexual partners have ever...

- Told you that you were a loser, a failure, or not good enough?
- Called you names like ugly, fat, crazy, or stupid?
- Insulted, humiliated, or made fun of you in front of others?
- Told you that no one else would want you?[48]

To be fair, and this should be emphasized, not all of the CDC questions were of this type. A full section dealt with questions that were indeed violent or even violently coercive or threatening, such as, "How many people have ever used physical force or threats" to have any type of sex.

But they also mix and match these types of questions, which are certainly legitimate, in a definition of rape or sexual violence with others and they label it the same way in the section titled "Sexual Violence."

Consider these additional questions:

How many people have ever...

- Harassed you while you were in a public place in a way that made you feel unsafe?
- Kissed you in a sexual way? Remember, we are only asking about things that you didn't want to happen.
- Fondled or grabbed your sexual body parts?

Who among us has not had at least one of these things happen? To get personal for a moment, I remember kissing a girl on the playground in third grade—and it was a surprise to both of us. Did she want it to happen? As I recall, however, she did not shun me afterward and indeed, was more friendly. Was this sexual *violence*?

I was also struck in a personal way, by this question—*making someone else look at or participate in sexual photos or movies.* In a candid moment with a woman in her 60s, she related how her husband showed her previously taken pictures of herself in her swimsuit. She did not want to look at them, but he said that she looked real good. She did not think so. She looked at the pictures anyway. Then he requested that she put on her swimsuit. She did not want to do that either and mildly objected, but then, she said to herself and him, "Oh well, if that's what you want. . ."

We are now all sexually violent criminals in some way, aren't we? At least, according to the CDC we are, if such behavior is classified as being part of the realm of "violence." However, we can expect that at least some will use the data and the definition to indicate and even more chillingly, indict all boys and men who initiate any kind of sexual behavior.

Coercion and Reproductive Health

It must be appreciated that the CDC survey did ask questions that simply had never been asked before in a large nationally representative survey—despite the conflation of violence with other types of behavior. In the section on violence by an intimate partner, we note here one of these areas, which is not violence, but can be accurately labeled as a type of sexual coercion:

Approximately 8.6% (or an estimated 10.3 million) of women in the United States reported ever having an intimate partner who tried to get them pregnant when they did not want to, or refused to use a condom, with 4.8% having had an intimate partner who

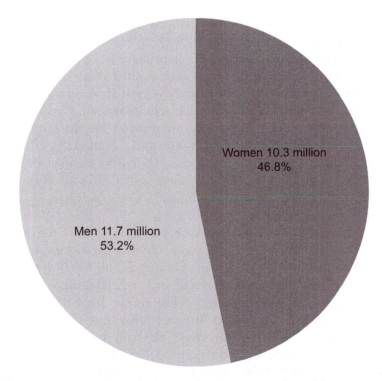

Graph 2.2   NISVS—Control of Reproductive or Sexual Health

tried to get them pregnant when they did not want to, and 6.7% having had an intimate partner who refused to wear a condom.

Approximately 10.4% (or an estimated 11.7 million) of men in the United States reported ever having an intimate partner who tried to get them pregnant when they did not want to or tried to stop them from using birth control, with 8.7% having had an intimate partner who tried to get pregnant when they did not want to or tried to stop them from using birth control and 3.8% having had an intimate partner who refused to wear a condom.[49]

Thus, there were more men who were victims of this type of sexually coercive behavior than were women for two out of the three measurements in the CDC survey (see Graph 2.2).[50]

Different Sentencing Standards

It is, unfortunately, nearly impossible to compare the sentences of male sexual offenders with female sexual offenders in a comprehensive and complete manner. On average, female offenders for *all* categories of crime receive lighter sentences than do men, according to the Department of Justice: "For each category of offense, women received shorter average maximum sentences than men. For property offenses, female prisoners had a mean sentence 42 months shorter than men, for drug offenses, 18 months shorter: and for violent offenses, 39 months shorter."[51] This result is indicative that female sexual assault offenders are likely to receive less prison time than males for the same type of offense. Overall, crime by women is increasing. Nationally, from 1993 through 2002, while overall crime was falling, the number of women arrested rose from 14 percent according to the FBI's Uniform Crime Report. In the same period, the number of men arrested fell by 5.9 percent.[52]

We might examine an anecdotal case, however, and ask the question, would a man in the same circumstances receive a harsher sentence?

In Bethlehem, New Jersey, Katrina Onufer, 26, hit her boyfriend with a hammer, stabbed him with knives and scissors, and disfigured his penis by biting, squeezing, and bruising it. The couple lived together at her mother's home. Assistant District Attorney Jacqueline Taschner said, "It looked like the guy had been tortured." She said the man weighed 300 pounds at the beginning of the relationship, but weighed only 70 pounds at the end of it. He was even punished for failing to clean up his own blood in a timely manner.

Onufer was convicted in 2004 of two counts of involuntary deviate sexual intercourse and single counts of aggravated assault, simple assault, and recklessly endangering another person. Her defense attorney argued that biting does not constitute sex, so the deviate sexual intercourse conviction should have been dropped.

In New Jersey, the deviate sexual intercourse conviction carries a standard range of four to five years in prison. The aggravated assault standard range is 22 months to 3 years.

Onufer got nine months in prison.[53]

In Missouri, the appeals court flatly rejected labeling a woman as a violent sexual predator, saying there was little evidence proving that women convicted of sex crimes are likely to become repeat offenders. Angela Coffel was the only woman in Missouri being held indefinitely as a violent sexual predator, after pleading guilty to the charges of sodomy against her two teenage brothers. She served five years in prison, but the state petitioned the court to keep her in prison, saying they had witnesses to prove that Coffel had "absolutely no control" over her sexual predatory behavior. The appeals court rejected that argument on gender grounds, the state Attorney General says the court's ruling created a gender double standard.[54] Coffel was released.

Little Research

In one sense, the Missouri court of appeals might be right, citing the fact of "little evidence." The research on female sexual offenders of any type is very limited.

Jacqueline Helfgott, a criminal research professor at Seattle University says, "There is a tendency among researchers, most of whom are men, to believe that women aren't capable of these types of crimes. We automatically think of sex offender as male. That sort of stops the exploration into research on females."[55]

Reactions and Effects

In *Sexual Coercion in Dating Relationships*,[56] researchers David and Cindy Struckman-Johnson find that there is a mixed bag of reactions by men to sexual coercion by women: "Equal numbers of men rated their reactions as bad and as good." They contend that four factors influence men's responses: "(1) the degree to which the advance violates his sexual standards, (2) the level of force used by the woman (3) the degree to which the woman is sexually desirable or creates sexual arousal by her actions, and (4) the extent to which a romantic relationship with the woman justifies the act."

The researchers concluded that low-force encounters with female sexual coercion resulted in few negative effects. However, "Actual male victims reported high levels of negative impact for incidents involving physical force or restraint by the woman." As might be expected, there was greater negative reactions to all types of sexual coercion by women when the man did not know the woman well: "The most conclusive finding of the study is that a majority of the men had a negative reaction to the idea of being pinned down for a sexual interaction by a woman whom they had only known for two hours."

In other words, far from being total sexual dogs, men like women, look at the circumstances of such coercive acts. Low-force acts are not viewed very negatively. If they had been dating the other person, and knew them fairly well and they found the other person attractive, then it was OK. In one sense, for men, such low-force acts—touching of genitals, performing oral sex, or initiating intercourse even—in a situation where the woman uses physical force such as pushing the man down, was not viewed very negatively. It may be that men find such acts even pleasant or acceptable under these circumstances because the pressure of being the sexual initiator and the fear of rejection is no longer a factor.

The Ultimate Taboo

A survey of 2,500 adult British men found that 3 percent of these were sexually assaulted as an adult and in nearly half of these cases, the perpetrator was a woman. Dr. Michael King told *Reuters Health*[57] that "The idea of women as perpetrators is not one that is easily acceptable politically, but actually it is quite common . . . Very few of (these episodes) are ever reported to either police or other professionals, like doctors." Although this study remains one of the largest and perhaps the largest epidemiological study of nonconsensual sexual experiences of men, (not counting for the moment, the CDC survey) the researchers did note that a Los Angeles area survey of 1,480 adult men found that 7 percent were victims of nonconsensual sex after age 16. This survey, however, did not distinguish between acts committed by women and those by men.

The late, Dr. Malcolm George of Queen Mary and Westfield Medical College in Great Britain prepared a previously unpublished article especially for this book. We will use his wonderful investigative research in some detail here.

"Despite the considerable number of books that have been written about men, masculinity and the male condition in present day society, by both men and women from widely differing perspectives, there is not a hint of this reality. It is the abuse that no one wants to contemplate."[58]

Dr. George points out that in their paper "Sexual Molestation of Men by Women," Sarrel and Masters[59] are especially noteworthy research exceptions:

> Masters, in his work with Johnson, is an acknowledged world expert in the field of human sexuality. Their paper went on to cite papers which described cases of men sexually abused by women. These men were seen because of sexual dysfunction that emanated from their experience of sexual abuse by adult women or groups of adult women and men. Subsequently Masters published a paper specifically on male sexual dysfunction resulting from such abuse. The authors suggested that the incidence of male rape and sexual molestation of men is underestimated because of the reluctance of men to report such abuse.

A paper by Cindy Struckman-Johnson[60] is exceptional in that it particularly sought to look at male victims of sexually coercive women. The authors stated that most studies of sexual abuse had only examined women's experience or, if they had included male subjects, had only asked men the extent to which they were perpetrators, not victims. It was noted, however, a few other studies had found rates of forced sex for men as well as women students. Struckman-Johnson's own study reported that female and male students' reported rates of forced sex were 22% for the sample of women and 16% for men. With follow up interviews it was possible to ascertain the type of coercion used. 52% of male victims reported psychological tactics while 16% of the female victims reported only this tactic. When it came to physical force 55% of the women reported this, but so did 10% of the men. However, about a quarter of the male victims were forced into sex by a combination of psychological pressure and some form of physical coercion.

In another paper for the *Journal of Sex Research*,[61] the percentages of men and women reporting physical coercion were about equal (6.5% men vs 5.8% women) with about half as many men as women reporting the use of actual physical violence to force submission to sexual intercourse (1.4% vs 2.7%). . . .Clearly, while the few cases and studies are a miniscule catalogue compared to the wealth of evidence on sexual abuse and rape of women by men, they do begin to suggest that men can be sexually abused by women. In investigating the cases of husbands battered by their wives, the author[62] has also come across cases where the emotional and physical abuse of the husband had been supplemented by sexual abuse. . . . [Note: As the author of *Abused Men: The Hidden Side of Domestic Violence,* I have noted the same phenomena with many of the men I interviewed for that book. Indeed, it is because of those interviews and related research that it was recommended by Dr. George and professionals who suggested that this book should be written to focus exclusively on the subject of adult women who sexually abuse men in various ways]. . . . Any number of men who had experienced this type of battering reported that they often had their genitals attacked, not just as an effective attack strategy, but also as a humiliating and emasculating degradation. Some men, additionally reported that the violence became more sexual in nature and sexual acts or intercourse were violent and even sadistically forced on them as the ultimate symbol of domination and humiliation. . . .

To put all this in another context of consideration. Abuse by a woman against another woman is not as unique as many would think—the studies of abuse within lesbian relationships show that it can be comparable or more prevalent than in heterosexual relations. Part of that abuse is coercive forced sex—woman on woman. The extent to which sexual abuse is a component mirrors that of heterosexual relationships. . . . [Note: In a study reported in *Abused Men,* there is a graph of research[63] showing that 31% *of lesbian couples reported forced sex acts compared to 12% of gay men reporting forced sex acts)*]. . . . In one study,[64] it was asked if sex had been forced and whether a gun or knife had been inserted into the victim's vagina. Four percent of those who said they had experienced forced sex, had suffered this kind of act. Surely, that is not just abuse, that is sexual terror! It is the sort of act that the most reviled, repugnant, despicably violent women-hating male rapists commit, isn't it?

The problem is, however, that society wishes to close its eyes to the plight of men who are emotionally and physically abused by wives or female partners. It is too destructive of all our cozy patriarchal notions of men and women and male and female stereotypical roles; woman as victim, man as perpetrator, women as sexually pursued, man as sexual pursuer. Sexually aggressive women and sexually victimized abused men really turn all that completely inside out and upside down. It makes it all seem as if real men and real women might be equal after all! That's why it is the ultimate taboo. And why it is something more difficult to contemplate.

The ultimate taboo and how society in general, the media, men and women react to such events, whether it be harassment, coercion, stalking, sexual assaults and rape is examined in our concluding chapter as will the implications for policy, intervention and treatment.

CHAPTER 3

Stalking

Famous Cases

When it happens to a man, as with other forms of sexual abuse by women, stalking is often viewed as being funny. Television comedian David Lettermen made the crime a regular routine out of the stalking directed against him. His stalker, Margaret Ray, was convicted and served a year in prison and was also sentenced to a year in a psychiatric hospital. She once camped out on his tennis court and frequently intruded into his home. She eventually committed suicide in 1998.

Network television's Conan O'Brien also made jokes about his being stalked by a male former Catholic priest. There were no jokes about Dawnette Knight, the stalker of actor Michael Douglas. She had sent threats to Douglas's wife, actress Catherine Zeta-Jones, saying she was going to slice her up like meat on a bone. At the trial, Zeta-Jones said she nearly suffered a nervous breakdown because of the threats. It is interesting to note that Douglas played a character being stalked by a woman in the 1987 film *Fatal Attraction*. Douglas also played a male victim of sexual harassment in a later film, *Disclosure*.

In 1949, Eddie Waitkus, a 29-year-old first baseman for the Philadelphia Phillies, was lured to a hotel room and shot by Ruth Ann Steinhagen, a fan who had been obsessed with him for a number of years.[1] This may have been the inspiration for a key scene in the movie *The Natural*, starring Robert Redford, in which a young baseball player was shot but not killed by an obsessed female fan. Actors John Cusack and Brad Pitt have also been stalked by female fans.

A review of the most prominent celebrity stalkers by NBC News[2] was not intended to offer a gender comparison. A review, however, of the celebrities listed, from Jerry Lewis to Uma Thurman, John Lennon, Monica Seles, and more, finds that about 85 percent of those doing the stalking are men, not women.

What Is Stalking?

The crime of stalking is typically defined as the willful, malicious, and repeated following and harassing of another person that threatens his or her safety. The National Violence Against Women Survey further defined stalking as, "A course of conduct directed at a specific person that involves repeated visual or physical proximity, nonconsensual communication, or verbal, written or implied threats or a combination thereof that would cause a reasonable person to fear."[3] The state of California became, in 1990, the first to make stalking a criminal offense. Most states quickly followed suit.

Tjaden and Thoennes define stalking as harassing or threatening behavior that an individual engages in repeatedly, such as following a person, appearing at a person's home or place of business, making harassing phone calls, leaving written messages or objects, or vandalizing a person's property.[4] As in most cases, the legal definition of stalking varies in different jurisdictions but is understood by most to include repeatedly harassing a person by following them or laying in wait, vandalism, and surveillance. The National Center for Victims of Crime defines stalking as "a course of conduct directed at a specific person that could cause a reasonable person to feel fear."[5]

Types of Stalking

Several types of stalkers were identified by Mullen et al. (2000)[6] and have been generally accepted or added to by other researchers:

- **The Rejected Stalker**: This represents the largest class of stalkers. These people pursue stalking behaviors, particularly telephone harassment, after a relationship has ended. That relationship was typically romantic or intimate but might also involve a work-related relationship or a relationship even with relatives.
- **Intimacy Seekers**: The second largest group of stalkers. Perhaps the most persistent of all stalkers. The victim and them were "destined" or "meant" to be together. About half of these suffer from

a delusional disorder, the other half simply suffer from infatuations that they recognized were not returned by their love object, but still "insist(ed), with delusional intensity, on both the legitimacy and the eventual success of their quest."

- **Incompetent Stalker**: These types of stalkers are notable in particular because they are more likely to have stalked more than one person. They typically lack social skills but feel a sense of entitlement or deserving to have a relationship with their victim. Most often, their victims are in an intimate relationship with someone else.
- **Resentful Stalker**: These stalkers act because they somehow feel wronged by the victim and are using various stalking tactics to frighten and upset the victim.
- **Predatory and Unprovoked Stalker**: The rarest form of stalker. They spy on their victim in various ways and use stalking-type activity to plan an actual attack. They may or may not have a personal relationship with the victim. The motives may be political, for example, it may be to gain fame or someone else's approval, or they are simply out to cause harm.

How Many Female Stalkers Are There?

As with all the areas we are exploring in this book, the available research on females sexually abusing men is not as much in total volume when compared to the reverse. The issue of stalking is no exception.

Estimates range from *6 percent to 26 percent for all stalking incidents by women against men*.[7] It seems that the proportion of female stalkers in the celebrity world might mirror that of the general population. Our random celebrity counting list is not a scientific study, of course, but it is interesting that it came up with about 15 percent of the total being identified as female stalkers. "Lifetime risks of being the victim of stalking have been measured in the United States, Australia, and Great Britain, and *range from 8 to 15 percent for women and 2 to 4 percent for men* (emphasis added)."[8]

Langhinrichsen-Rohling et al. used the Unwanted Pursuit Behaviors Inventory (UPBI) to determine the prevalence of "former-intimate stalking-type" behaviors in an undergraduate population. This study finds no sex differences in overall UPBI scores of individuals who are the "dumpees." Females and males indicate that they engage in stalking acts to the same degree in their inventory responses.

Additionally, there are no sex differences in the number of unwanted pursuit behaviors (UPBs) experienced by those who initiated the break-up. "Males and females who had instigated the break-up were equally likely to be the victims of UPBs by their former-intimates, which included theft, physical harm and being followed." Interestingly, males were found to be the victims of cyber stalking by a former-intimate more than their female counterparts (Alexy et al., 2005). Mullen et al. (2001) also find that female stalkers are more likely to favor electronic stalking acts than physical acts, show the same propensity for threats, physical violence and property damage as male offenders, are more motivated to establish a love relationship with their victims and are likely to target men and women equally with their stalking behaviors.[9]

According to the National Violence Against Women Survey (1997), nearly 371,000 men are victimized by stalkers in the United States each year. One out of every 12 women will be stalked during her lifetime. One out of 45 men will be stalked during a lifetime, for a total of 1,006,970 women and 370,990 men who are stalked every year.[10]

The (2006) Supplemental Victimization Survey from the U.S. Department of Justice which was reported in 2009 found that "Males were as likely to report being stalked by a male as a female offender. *43% of male stalking victims stated that the offender was female* (emphasis added), while 41% of male victims stated that the offender was another male. Female victims of stalking were significantly more likely to be stalked by a male (67%) rather than a female (24%) offender."[11]

Davis, Coker, and Sanderson analyzed data from the National Violence Against Women survey: "With a criterion of being stalked on more than one occasion and being at least 'somewhat afraid,' 14.2% of women and 4.3% of men were victims. Among those stalked, 41% of women and 28% of men were stalked by an intimate partner. Women were more than 13 times more likely to be 'very afraid' of their stalker than men. *Negative health consequences of being stalked were similar for men and women* (emphasis added); those stalked were significantly more likely to report poor current health, depression, injury, and substance use."[12]

Rita Handrich, PhD is a licensed psychologist in the state of Texas, and a consultant with Keene Trial Consulting. Prior to joining the firm, she served as an expert witness, communications and organizational consultant, and psychotherapist. She points out in referencing the above study that it "only included victims/subjects who feared bodily harm from their stalkers. Realizing that men are less likely to report being fearful of woman due to the male masculine stereotype there was a small percentage of men who actively took part in the study; we can surmise that some men would not report being fearful of a woman due to fear of being harassed by other males thus making the actual percentage higher than what is reported in this study."[13]

Indeed, what questions are asked, how they are asked, and whether or not there was gender bias or blindness to possibly unique male concerns affects all research in this area. The National Violence Against Women Survey, as we have pointed out, contains flaws in failing to ask questions about intimate violence that more particularly might apply to men, such as failing to ask questions about scalding liquids and poison use, to give but a few examples. It is also criticized for "mixing" intimate crime and "general" crime. Generally, sociologists know that general crime surveys that might include asking information about burglary are more likely to lower the rate of reporting about family violence issues. Whether this fact would also contaminate in a sense the mixing of crimes such as rape and stalking (where it might be a stranger or non-intimate) in the Violence Against Women Survey is open to debate.

Handrich says her review of the literature reveals these conclusions:

- Male stalkers are more likely to be prosecuted than female stalkers.
- There appear to be *comparable rates of violence* [1 of 3 female stalkers will threaten and 1 of 4 will be violent toward the target or the target's property in equal measure]
- There was also a difference in what the researchers call the "primary pattern of pursuit." Female stalkers never used third parties to deliver their messages. They were more likely to fax, write letters, or send gifts or packages but less likely to make personal contact with the target or commit burglaries.
- Women stalkers were also more benign in their communications than were male stalkers. They were more likely to "just communicate" or "seek help" than the men but also "less insulting." Women made fewer threats (either implied or direct) and women were more likely than men to threaten the family or friends of the target (or even threaten to harm themselves). When women were violent, it was more likely to be predatory than emotionally driven. And women were more likely (much

more likely) to be violent if they were stalking a victim with whom they had a prior history of sexual intimacy.

In the peer-reviewed journal *Innovations in Clinical Neuroscience*,[14] Sara G. West, MD and Susan Hatters Friedman, MD, both from the Department of Psychiatry at University Hospitals, Case Western School of Medicine in Cleveland, Ohio, did a review of the available research on female stalkers. They cleverly titled the article, "These Boots Are Made for Stalking."

West and Hatters Friedman summarized the work of the relatively well-known researchers in the field but did find two lesser-known studies:

Battered Women Who Stalk

A study focusing on stalking and unwanted pursuit behavior perpetrated by 55 women residing in a battered women's shelter was published in 2006. A limitation of this study, as described by the authors, involved an inability to ask the subjects, due to the concerns of the shelter employees, about their motivations for perpetrating the stalking behavior.

The women, on average, were in their early 30s, were unemployed, and had children. The specific acts perpetrated by this group of women included begging the abuser not to leave, seeking information from others about the abuser, giving the abuser unwanted gifts, visiting the abuser unexpectedly, following the abuser, making a threat toward the abuser, or threatening suicide or self-harm. It was noted that, if these women had themselves previously been a victim of these behaviors, they were more likely to become a perpetrator of similar behavior. These women were more likely to form insecure attachments, suffer from depression, blame themselves for the abuse, and leave the shelter quickly compared to other women in the shelter who did not participate in stalking or unwanted pursuit behavior.

LAPD Study

In an effort to determine the degree of intimacy in the stalker-victim relationship, Palarea, et al., compared 135 intimate and 88 non-intimate stalkers investigated by the Los Angeles Police Department's Threat Management Unit. Women accounted for 22 percent of the sample. Unfortunately, despite a large amount of data collected on this group, not much of it was analyzed specifically by gender. Intimate stalkers were married to, engaged to, cohabited with, dated, or had a casual sexual relationship with the victim. The authors determined that women were somewhat more likely to participate in non-intimate stalking (57.1%) when compared to intimate stalking. This differed from the men, who were more likely to be suspects in the intimate stalking cases (65.5%).

West and Hatters Friedman sum up what they found in their concluding statement: "Female stalkers tend to target people that they know, and they are capable of threatening their victims and even becoming violent. We must be cautious not to underestimate women's potential for violence secondary to a gender bias."

Meanwhile, a 2009 Department of Justice National Crime Victimization Survey found:

- 3.4 Million Stalker Victims in a Year
- During a 12-month period an estimated 14 in every 1,000 persons age 18 or older were victims of stalking.
- About half (46%) of stalking victims experienced at least one unwanted contact per week, and 11% of victims said they had been stalked for 5 years or more.
- The risk of stalking victimization was highest for individuals who were divorced or separated—34 per 1,000 individuals.
- Women were at greater risk than men for stalking victimization; however, women and men were equally likely to experience harassment.
- Male (37%) and female (41%) stalking victimizations were equally likely to be reported to the police.
- Approximately 1 in 4 stalking victims reported some form of cyber stalking such as e-mail (83%) or instant messaging (35%).
- 46% of stalking victims felt fear of not knowing what would happen next.
- More than half of the stalking victims lost 5 or more days of work for due to fear of their safety or dealing with legal attempts to remedy the situation.[15]

Peter Main of Houston, Texas should have been fearful when Toni Jo Silvey, an ex-lover called him 146 times in a 24-hour timeframe, vandalized his home with eggs, broke several windows, and started a blog dedicated to describing the details of their breakup.[16] On Tuesday,

October 11, 2011, Silvey was arrested and charged with felony stalking. In the state of Texas, Penal Code §42.072 states that a person can be charged with stalking if they cause a reasonable person to fear bodily injury or death for himself or herself or that an offense will be committed against the person's property. When Silvey egged Main's house, she took pictures and posted them on her Facebook page! Apparently, she did not think she would be treated as a criminal for harassing and destroying Main's property. The stalking had been going on for years (2009–2011), but Main told police he had been reluctant to file charges against her because "he is afraid of angering (her) further."[17]

From England, the BBC reported another remarkable stalking case—that of a woman who terrorized a doctor with texts, emails, and phone calls:

> Jurors heard Maria Marchese, 45, hounded Dr. Jan Falkowski, 45, for three years and falsely accused him of rape.
>
> Marchese, of Bow, east London, also sent death threats to Dr. Falkowski's then-fiancee Deborah Pemberton.
>
> At Southwark Crown Court, she was found guilty of harassment and charges of threats to kill. Marchese was also convicted of perverting the course of justice after the three-week trial.
>
> As well as sending messages declaring undying love for the psychiatrist she warned Ms Pemberton that she would be "burnt down in her wedding dress" if she dared marry him.
>
> Eventually the couple called off their wedding and separated.
>
> Marchese also falsified DNA evidence against the doctor by retrieving one of his condoms from a rubbish bin to back up claims that he raped her, the court heard.
>
> Judge John Price told her: "You got into their lives in the most extraordinary way and found out about their day-to-day existence." "You have gone to the most extraordinary lengths of accusing him of rape . . . that could have left him with a prison sentence. You have terrorised them. . . ."
>
> In a statement released after the verdict Dr Falkowski said he was relieved his "nightmare" was finally over.
>
> But he also said he had been the victim of numerous failures in the legal system and called for anonymity in rape cases to extend to the accused until the trial.
>
> As a result of Marchese's claims he was charged with rape in 2004 but cleared in 2005.
>
> He said he hoped the case would ensure stalking victims are taken seriously in the future.

"I hope that by reading about our harrowing experiences of being stalked, other victims of stalking and of rape allegations will feel that they are not alone," he added.[18]

Differences and Similarities

We borrow heavily here from the conclusions of researchers Meloy and Boyd writing in the *Journal of the American Academy of Psychiatry and the Law*[19] and the prior work of Purcell et al.[20] in the *Journal of American Psychiatry*. These researchers, in particular, have been conducting groundbreaking work into the subject of male and female differences and similarities related to stalking. We summarize some of their conclusions here based on their own original research, but more importantly, drawing from the work of all those published in the field:

- Female stalkers are more persistent than male stalkers given certain motivations.
- Female stalkers appear to be similar to male stalkers in age and relationship status: most appear to be single women in their mid-30s.
- A history of failed sexual pair bonds appears to mark both male and female stalkers.
- Education and IQ appear to be higher among female stalkers than female criminals in general, a finding that has been replicated in male samples.
- Delusional disorder has been shown to be more frequent in females than in males in civil mental health settings.
- Most male stalkers knew their victims and the most common prior relationship was sexual intimacy. Males tend to be stalked by female acquaintances and strangers, not by prior sexual intimates. This may support a *theory* that those female stalkers are motivated to establish intimacy with their victims, whereas male stalkers are attempting to maintain intimacy with their former partners.
- The most frequently prohibited act in stalking laws, following the victim, is engaged in less often by females than by males. They appear to be creatively aggressive in more covert ways: they intrude on the victim's associates, vandalize property, use surveillance, break and enter, and steal the victim's possessions. All of these patterns do not risk a direct physical confrontation with the male victim, at least for the moment.

- Stalking victims were most likely to be slightly older male acquaintances; but if the victim was a prior sexual intimate of the female stalker, her risk of being violent toward him exceeded 50 percent. Unlike male stalkers who often pursue their victims to restore intimacy, these female stalkers often pursued their victims to establish intimacy. Common emotions and motivations included anger, obsessional thoughts, and rage at abandonment, loneliness, dependency, jealousy, and perceived betrayal.
- What motivates female stalkers? Anger and hostility were reported in two-thirds of the females, as it was in a majority of male stalkers. Perhaps unwanted following is more overtly aggressive, therefore more likely to be a male stalking behavior.
- More male stalkers reported a history of criminal offenses. Higher rates of substance abuse were also noted among the male stalkers, but the psychiatric status of the groups did not otherwise differ. The duration of stalking and the frequency of associated violence were equivalent. The nature of the prior relationship with the victim differed, with female stalkers more likely to target professional contacts and less likely to harass strangers. Female stalkers were also more likely than male stalkers to pursue victims of the same gender. The majority of female stalkers were motivated by the desire to establish intimacy with their victim, whereas men showed a broader range of motivations.

Purcell et al. have a concluding statement that is worthy of particular attention: "Female and male stalkers vary according to the motivation for their pursuit and their choice of victim. A female stalker typically seeks to attain a close intimacy with her victim, who usually is someone previously known and frequently is a person cast in the professional role of helper. *While the contexts for stalking may differ by gender, the intrusiveness of the behaviors and potential for harm does not* (emphasis added)."

In other words, there are differences between the genders in the style by which they commit certain acts, but the substantive effects of their acts are likely to be similar. Purcell, Pathé, and Mullen comment:

Contrary to popular assumptions, this study found that female stalkers are no less likely than their male counterparts to threaten their victims or attack their person or property. Male stalkers were more likely, however, to progress from explicit threats to physical assaults on the victim. The methods of harassment were largely equivalent between the groups, the exceptions being telephone calls (favored by all but one female stalker) and following (preferred by male stalkers). The tenacity male and female stalkers apply to their quest is also strikingly similar. Thus, while the contexts for stalking vary between men and women, the intrusiveness of the conduct and its potential for harm does not. There is no reason to presume that the impact of being stalked by a female would be any less devastating than that of a man. . . .

Women undoubtedly are the predominant victims of the crime of stalking, but it is important to recognize that in a significant minority of stalking cases, women are the perpetrators. Female stalkers are typically socially isolated individuals with high rates of mental illness and characterological disturbance. Although driven in some instances by resentment or retaliation for perceived hurts, the majority are motivated by a desire to establish an intimate relationship with the victim.[21]

False Stalking

Psychologist Michael G. Conner is a member of the American Psychological Association and board certified in traumatic stress, emergency crisis response, and school crisis response. In an online article on stalking, he takes a somewhat different view of the phenomena. He does describe it a manner that is similar to those by other researchers and experts, as we have presented here. Somewhat rarely, however, his article features some cautions about false reports or beliefs that one is being stalked:

> Nearly 90% of all college students who break up will engage in what is called "unwanted pursuit behavior." Pursuit behavior includes writing notes, giving gifts, making phone calls, contacting friends, following the person or intruding in their life. This can border and easily cross the line and become an obsession. What researchers find interesting is that pursuit behavior is normal. If Jane dissolves a relationship with Bob, then it is very common for Bob to pursue Jane as a means to restore the relationship. Researchers call this a "relationship repair mechanism." Some people and even the courts mistakenly call this stalking. . . . Researchers have found that about 1 out of 24 people who are convinced they are being stalked actually aren't. And about 1 out of 49 people who are being stalked actually don't believe they are. Now here is where it all gets interesting. Some people who claim to be stalked suffer from what

has been called "false stalking syndrome." This syndrome (a pattern of behavior) confuses the public, the courts, law enforcement and even the friends of the so-called victim . . . Women with false stalking syndrome will go to the police, ministers, friends and others to gain support, friendship and escape from problems in their life. It has not been established whether or not men have this syndrome. Women with this condition are typically dramatic, sexually provocative, live chaotic lives, suffer repeated relationship failures, have financial problems and have very dysfunctional histories usually involving drug or alcohol use. They also have histories of being stalked or know people who have been stalked. Any person who repeatedly places their self in proximity of a person they claim is stalking them is likely to suffer from false stalking syndrome or may be involved in false crime reporting.[22]

Conner contends that this aspect of stalking is limited to women almost exclusively, and that women with this syndrome actually engage in stalking tactics themselves by going to their target's place of employment, home, church, and so on, but still claim to be the stalking victim.

I do not always agree with the conclusions of Charles Corry, PhD, of the Equal Justice Foundation in Colorado, who has long maintained a web presence regarding issues affecting males. I do appreciate, however, his analysis here in regards to questions from the National Violence Against Women Survey, which we previously mentioned. He points out that the Survey asked these stalking questions:

Not including bill collectors, telephone solicitors, or other salespeople, has anyone, male or female ever . . .

- Followed or spied on you?
- Sent you unsolicited letters or written correspondence?
- Made unsolicited phone calls to you?
- Stood outside your home, school, or workplace?
- Showed up at places you were even though he or she had no business being there?
- Left unwanted items for you to find?
- Tried to communicate in other ways against your will?
- Vandalized your property or destroyed something you loved?

Respondents who answered yes to one or more of these questions were asked whether anyone had ever done any of these things to them on more than one occasion and whether they felt frightened or feared bodily harm as a result of these behaviors. Only respondents who reported being victimized on more than one occasion, and who were very frightened or feared bodily harm were counted as stalking victims.[23]

Corry contends that these questions lend themselves to a variety of scenarios that can now be defined as stalking:

- You call a girl up that you met asking for a date. She says she is busy. You see her somewhere again and say hi. She smiles, so you try for another date. No go. Try again and it must be *"stalking."* . . .
- You have a disagreement and she never wants to see you again. You send roses with a note. No response. You try calling a couple of times. That must be *"stalking"* as well.
- You write her a letter or email saying you're sorry, and you would like to make up. You work in the same building and you leave the letter on her chair at work or send the email to her. You must be *"stalking"* her. *Sending a letter or email can now be considered a crime!* . . .
- You've broken up. After you try calling her a couple of times, you run into some friends of hers and ask how she is doing. Could it be you are spying on her? . . .

Most people would regard such events as well within the normal course of human affairs. The path to true romance is filled with potholes but now we've made it a crime. *Is that wise?* Remember, in such cases proof is not required, a female *"victim"* is believed without reservation or question, and hearsay is admissible. Of course it isn't considered possible that the *"victim"* could be paranoid or psychotic. And her *"fear"* must be considered *"reasonable"* regardless of the actual circumstances. How likely is it she might use such charges as revenge for some real or imagined wrong you may have done her? Maybe you deal with females on another planet than the one I live on, but such raw, naked power to destroy **will** be used with evil intent here.[24]

Corry also mentions behavior that is rarely considered or named as part of a stalking by researchers, therapists, courts, or law enforcement. He correctly points out, however, that this kind of tactic is not unusual, whatever it might be called. More aptly, it might be called *Set-up Stalking.*

A husband and wife are divorced and he receives child visitation. There is also a restraining order issued against him because he has been accused of domestic violence or it has been issued based on her fear that she might be physically harmed. The order prohibits him from coming within a specified distance of her. He arrives at her home, to return the children from a weekend visitation, he gets out of the car to open the door for them. She calls the police and he is arrested. This scenario is indeed an actual case that I am familiar with and was verified with an attorney who filed court papers on behalf of the husband. Corry reports incidents in which women get the restraining order, follow the man with their cell phone in hand, and then, when he is within the required distance that would trigger a violation, she calls the police to have him arrested.

Advice for Men

Dr. Tara J. Palmatier is a psychologist who specializes in issues affecting men and has a website with articles and a Comments section. She wrote an article called "Female Stalkers—What Is Stalking and Can Men Be Stalked by Women?"[25] The article is an excellent summation of the research, but she also offers some direct advice:

> Stalking and other forms of harassment are criminal behaviors, whether the perpetrator is a male or female. Stalking typically occurs after a break up, although, it can also occur at the onset and throughout the course of the relationship (for example, does your wife hack into your email?) **Many men view stalking behavior in women as normal female insecurity, jealousy and/or possessiveness. These are *not* normal behaviors; they're abnormal and abusive behaviors.** They're indicative of an individual who has a lack of boundaries, a shaky grasp on reality and sociopathic tendencies (i.e., no empathy for how her victims are feeling and the belief that only her needs, feelings and desires matter).
>
> If you're beginning to date someone and she displays stalking/ harassment behaviors, it should be a huge red flag (i.e., you need to stop seeing her). If your wife or girlfriend is guilty of these behaviors, you need to understand that this is abuse and it's wrong. If your ex-wife is stalking/harassing you and/or your new girlfriend/ wife/family, you need to take legal measures to protect yourself and your loved ones. The reason so many women get away with these

behaviors is because not enough people take them seriously. Our society will begin to take this issue seriously if we start prosecuting women who engage in these behaviors—just like we do with male offenders.

Perhaps some men aren't physically afraid of their female stalkers, but that doesn't make their behavior any less criminal. Being stalked and/or the target of a harassment campaign can be incredibly stressful, irritating and frustrating. Law abiding citizens—including male law abiding citizens—have a right to the peaceful enjoyment of their lives free from harassment.

[Men] who find themselves the victim of a female stalker often confront indifference and skepticism from law enforcement and other helping agencies. Not infrequently, **male victims allege that their complaints have been trivialized or dismissed, some victims being told that they should be "flattered" by all the attention.**

Victimization studies indicate that women are seldom prosecuted for stalking offenses, with criminal justice intervention most likely to proceed in those cases involving a male suspect accused of stalking a woman. The available evidence suggests that **stalking by women has yet to be afforded the same degree of seriousness attached to harassment perpetrated by men.** This is so, despite any empirical evidence that women are any less intrusive or persistent in their stalking or pose any less of a threat (physical or otherwise) to their victims.

Further advice on actions the stalking victim might take comes from a review of the research presentation by Doris Hall, PhD at California State University, Bakersfield. There is even a sample letter one could present to a stalker: "No matter what you may have assumed till now, and no matter for what reason you assumed it, I have no romantic interest in you whatsoever. I never will. I expect that knowing this, you'll put your attention elsewhere, which I understand, because that is what I intend to do."

Hall adds some critical advice that may not be easily considered at first by the victim: "A Critical part of risk management is frequent and effective communication. If the police or employer takes action which might anger or embarrass the stalker the target needs to be advised, or the stalking victim is put at further risk." She adds these further steps for risk management:

- Document, document, document
- Maintain log of all contact

- Change daily schedule and routes
- Alert trusted neighbors, coworkers, family, and friends
- Cease all contact with stalker
- Code word on all utilities
- Have a safety plan
- Carry a disposable camera and a video camera

Further advice for victims of stalking include not only taking the obvious step of changing phone numbers to be given out only to trusted friends and family, but also keeping the old one that the harasser may have so that a record of harassing calls can be kept. The same with emails and text messages—keep them so that a record is made for law enforcement and prosecutors, but never respond. Victims should make sure that work calls are screened by others and anonymous packages should never be accepted. Buying a dog, taking a course in self-defense, changing locks, using a passport instead of a driver's license for identification, and not accepting mail at a home address are other recommended steps. There are also a number of books currently available with useful information about general privacy protection that can be applied to stalking situations. More than anything else, victims should not give harassers the one thing they want the most—personal attention.

A Man Tells His Story

In her Shrink 4 Men website, Dr. Palmatier received about 40 comments on her article and men told their stories of stalking. This one is typical, but especially instructive as to the details of what the official reaction was to the incidents:

The day after the breakup the phone calls started. At first, it was more the begging for me to "take her back" type. After 40–50 no's then the harassing calls started. If I didn't unplug the phone they would continue through the ENTIRE night. I blocked her number, so she would go buy prepaid cell phones. I changed my number to unlisted & somehow she would get the new number.

It didn't take long to escalate into threats against my life. My tires were slashed, my windshield was smashed three times causing my insurance company to drop my coverage. I reported it to the police but they needed evidence that SHE was the one doing it. She started calling my friends, my workplace, my family etc. My band did a show & she showed up. The bouncers had to remove her. This became a HUGE nightmare.

Finally one night she shows up at my door, drunk (with her 2 kids in the car) banging on my door at 2 AM threatening to 'burn my house down, kill me & cut my balls off' The police showed up but since her dad was a county sheriff they let him pick her up & drive everybody home. NO CHARGES were filed. They told me "well, she's a woman, you can protect yourself & if we take her to jail we have to take the kids into custody, so we don't want to do that."

Less than a week later she did THE EXACT SAME THING! Once again the police refused to arrest her despite the fact that anti-stalking laws were on the books. 911 Had her on tape screaming threats against my life & property through the door. All the police were willing to do was to make her "promise" to leave me alone. I asked for a restraining order to back that up & they refused. Why? They didn't want to give "this poor lady" (their exact words) a record of any kind. They further stated that I must have done something pretty bad for her to react like this.

But wait it gets even better. The next day I talked to a lawyer & filed an order of protection against her. Well this REALLY set her off. The following Sunday morning the police were at MY door with a warrant for MY arrest for, get this, domestic assault charges. She filed a claim with the Co. Sheriff (the one her dad worked for) that I had assaulted her the previous night. This crazy woman even went as far as to scar her own face. I have no idea how except that she either had somebody hit her or did it herself. I was arrested, led away in handcuffs, had to post bail & hire a lawyer to defend myself.

Fortunately for me, the night she claimed I did this my band was doing a show in front of thousands of screaming fans & witnesses. She wasn't the sharpest knife in the drawer. BUT I still had to post $500 bail, pay a lawyer $1,500 to defend these charges, pay a P I another $1500 to get witness statements that my band was at a show. I was suspended from without pay from work pending the outcome of this. My boss didn't believe the charges but I was a bonded employee so they couldn't take the chance.

I was cleared & demanded that this crazy woman be arrested for filing a false charge. The cops refused AGAIN!!! It took me & my lawyer going to the DA's office demanding she be charged. I was lucky in that I got a female DA who HATED stalkers. Her husband had to deal with an ex-wife like such so she knew how crazy & dangerous they can get. She filed the charges, and had her arrested. When the court date came the judge (who was a friend of her family) threw out the case. No explanation, just tossed it.

These last incidents did stop the stalking however & I have had no contact with her since. But let's review. What did she learn from this? She learned that she can file false charges against somebody who dumped her. The poor sap has to pay thousands in bail & lawyer fees, P I cost etc. & she has ABSOLUTELY NO consequences. So my advice to anybody in a similar situation would be contact police the DAY it starts. Even if they won't do anything then MAKE THEM file a report so you have a record of the behavior.

This was a nightmare that took over 6 months to play out.

Cyber Stalking

It is a brave new world and cyber stalking has heartily embraced it. Hacking, viruses that monitor personal computers, hidden cameras and microphones, and GPS tracking have all been added to arsenal. In some sense, the "old" style of sending abusive emails, malicious emails and similar postings on websites, comment boards, message boards or signing up the target to unwanted online services, or sending messages pretending to be the other person, are in danger of being eclipsed. Being "followed" on Twitter, in this context, certainly takes on a new meaning.

The spreading of malicious rumors or simply lying about another person on the net is certainly a big part of cyber stalking. It is the apparent anonymity of the net that can encourage such behavior. Telling another person to their face or even over the phone that so-and-so is really a pedophile and should not be coaching children (an actual case) is relatively easy to do anonymously on the net. Creating a fake Facebook page, pretending to be another person who is the target is becoming another frequently used method. Dr. Emma Short is a psychologist who has published research on stalking, and says, "My research has shown that everybody has an idea of the rules of the internet, but the problem is that everyone's idea is slightly different. I gave a lecture recently where one girl said that she was considering calling the police because her ex-boyfriend had posted graphic photos of her on Facebook, and then another student said she had just split up with her boyfriend and had done the exact same thing. She said it was fine because 'he had it coming.'"[26]

Meanwhile, there are websites and posts that actually encourage and teach young women how to cyber stalk more effectively. It is called "Creepin'" instead of stalking, though even the blogs on CollegeCandy admit that is what it is:

> Facebook can turn even the most confident girl into a crazy stalker. Whether it's clicking rapidly through photo albums and tagged pictures or checking out every single girl who posts on your random hook-up's wall, we've all been there. And that's OK. It's not like we're sitting in a windowless van outside some-one's house for hours, watching their every move. No, we're just reading what they wanted us to read. No privacy settings, no problem!
>
> But while creepin' on The Book is totes acceptable, there are some things that just aren't. So if you're so-bored-you-want-to-die at your summer job, or even if you're just obsessed with finding out which of your long lost high school peers has gotten knocked up—if you want to keep your creeping under wraps remember these few things when you go on a stalking expedition.[27]

More Male than Female Cyber Stalking Victims?

A United Kingdom online survey by the Network for Surviving Stalk-ing and conducted by Emma Short, a psychologist at the University of Bedfordshire, found that about 35 percent of those who responded and said they were stalked using online technology were males.[28] While the percentage is correct, however, the number of participants in the sur-vey was overwhelmingly female (240 women compared to 109 men). Short told the *Daily Mail* newspaper that Facebook makes it easier: "Facebook makes stalking more acceptable and removes the aspect of physical fear. . . . Women who would not be able to overpower men physically can have a go at them online."[29]

The limitations of voluntary online surveys even by respected soci-ologists are obvious. More reliable perhaps are online security experts who make preventing hacking, identity theft, and other crimes their business.

Garlik is an online major security firm also based in the United King-dom. They found using a variety of methods, including modeling of major crime reports, police reports, and their own client-based meth-odology that 394,000 men were online stalking victims compared to 135,000 women.[30] That's about *3 percent of men compared to 1 percent of female victims* in the United Kingdom.

Why is there such a marked difference in the results? We appreciate the Garlik statement about measuring this type of crime: "There are **no** (emphasis added) comprehensive public statistics kept on victims of online harassment or cyber stalking by ISP's, government or police." Garlik used a variety of methods: "Books, journal articles 'grey' literature (such as conference proceedings and newspapers), official publications. . . .Where possible, statistics were derived from interview surveys. Such interviews can provide a better reflection of the true extent of cybercrime because they encompass crimes that are not reported to the police." There is little reason to suspect that the results of a similar type of investigation in the United States would reveal dissimilar results.

Garlik's research found that men are not as careful as women on the internet. Criminologist Emily Finch at the legal research firm 1871 Ltd. was quoted as saying that "men typically guard themselves less than women" on the internet and therefore are more easily exposed to online crime. Some indicators of this are that men outnumber women in several key categories:

Give out phone number on social networking sites: Men = 20% Women = 14%
Post Residence address: Men = 16% Women = 13%
Detailed description of achievements and lives: Men = 16% Women = 8%

The researchers found that although more than 80 percent of cyber stalking cases go unreported to police, part of the reason may be that fully a quarter of the male victims felt that the police would not take their complaint seriously, while 6 percent said they would not report it because of fear. Twenty-one percent of all respondents, male and female, felt that it was due to their own lack of care on the internet in posting personal information.

Tom Illube, Garlik's chief executive, says their research demonstrates the "Need for all consumers to be cautious about the kinds of information they provide online and to be vigilant about monitoring their online identity. It dispels a common stereotype that men are unlikely to fall victim to cyber stalking."

It does seem to happen and more often than one might assume. If it is true that more women participate in cyber stalking than men, it may be because following ex-boyfriends on the web or harassing them is simply easier to do than the "old" methods of physically following someone or staking out their residence.

It would be an interesting article, perhaps in a woman's magazine, to ask readers' opinions on whether women are more likely to engage in this activity and why. The editor of *Northwest Women Magazine* will likely not have that opportunity, as reported by KXLY television in Spokane, Washington, in a copyrighted story:

> The editor of Northwest Woman Magazine, published in Spokane, is wrapped up in an identity theft case. The Spokane County Prosecutor's Office is charging Charity Doyl with identity theft, theft and cyber stalking. Northwest Woman Magazine is published out of offices on Spokane's South Hill and reaches about 40,000 people. The editor, Charity Doyl, is involved in an identity theft and cyber stalking case that reaches back to late 2009. In court documents obtained by KXLY her accuser is also her ex-boyfriend, Martin Dow of Glen Dow Academy. Dow told officers that after the two broke up he began receiving threatening and harassing emails from Doyl.
>
> The threatening emails included an eVite invitation to a Super Bowl party. The title of the eVite reads: DON'T PISS ME OFF—I HAVE YOUR EMAIL LIST. The email addresses she is alluding to, according to court documents, are the thousands of email address contacts Dow has as a business owner. Months after the threats and stalking took place, Dow found a new girlfriend, and court documents say, the harassment resurfaced.
>
> This time, Dow told police, Doyl used his credit card or credit card number to rack up over $3500 worth of Russian goods and send them to his office. According to court documents, on May 18th 2010 Dow received a shipment of fresh Russian fish. The deliveries continued that day, and he received caviar and Russian magazines and newspapers. Coincidentally or not, Dow's new girlfriend was a Russian immigrant.[31]

Dow gave this statement to the station: "There has been no threat to our livelihood, nor to me personally, more potentially onerous than false and malicious information posted or threatened to be posted on electronic networks."

Responses to Stalking

In "Female Stalkers and Their Victims" in the *Journal of American Academy of Psychiatry and the Law,*[32] we find out how the victims responded to *all types* of stalking attacks. The authors' list of the most common result, to least common, is instructive. We find that a majority did take steps to document the evidence, and somewhat surprisingly, the next most likely reaction was to obtain a temporary restraining order. The third action, taken in what was called "the team approach," was to talk to a variety of other people and get their help, such as friends, law enforcement, and mental health professionals. Other methods used, in order, were to change habit patterns; report to the police; increase security; change phone numbers, change address, carry a weapon; seek psychotherapy, and change the place of employment.

Consequences of Stalking

A review of the literature on what happens to stalking victims was presented by Doris Hall, PhD, at California State University, Bakersfield:

- Anxiety (83%)
- Sleep disturbances (74%)
- Overwhelming Powerlessness (75%)
- Flashbacks/Intrusive recollections (55%)
- Fatigue (55%)
- Weight fluctuation (48%)
- Headaches (47%)
- Reduced social outings (70%)
- Reduction in work/school attendance (53%)
- Relocation (39%)
- Change in workplace, school, or career (37%)[33]

It Never Ends

Mullen, Pathé, and Purcell, in their book, *Stalkers and Their Victims,* find that stalking is a different kind of crime and has a pernicious effect on victims:

Stalking victims are subjected to persistent repetitive trauma, as opposed to most other victims of crime and other isolated traumatic events. Not only do the stalkers repeated intrusions represent a loss of control for the victim, but the often ineffectual response of the criminal justice system and other helping agencies violates the stalking victims of living in a fair and safe society and crushes their expectations of regaining control.

These victims live in a state of persistent threat with associated symptoms that may far outlive the actual duration of the harassment.[34]

Different Consequences for Men and Women?

There are a few studies that looked into the gender difference issue. Some samples of our review are presented here. The first is from the *Journal of Interpersonal Violence*: "In a majority of mental health scales, women score poorer than men, and a higher percentage of women fulfill criteria for a current mental disorder and used psychotropic medication. However, effects of gender decrease to a non-significant level when stalking victimization is entered into the respective models. Furthermore, associations of stalking victimization with poor mental health, psychosocial functioning, and use of medication are largely comparable across gender."[35]

The *Journal of Consulting and Clinical Psychology*[36] adds that, "Results revealed no meaningful interactive effects of gender and interpersonal aggression on outcomes, once lifetime exposure to aggressive events was adequately taken into account. These findings argue against theories of female victims' greater vulnerability to pathological outcomes, instead linking risk to exposure history."

Trends

It appears then, that there is very little difference in the *effects* of what happens to stalking victims, whether they are male or female. This mirrors the results from our previously published work on all types of intimate partner violence. Both males and females engage in a huge variety of stalking behaviors. The *types* of stalking behavior carried out do seem to vary with gender, but the overall differences are slight. Certainly, the best available evidence so far indicates that more males than females engage in stalking activity, with the exception of cyber stalking. Given the phenomenal and continued growth of social networking sites and the internet in general, we can expect the female proclivity for this type of attack to continue at a rapid pace.

Lots of Money but Little Help

There is small (all volunteer) group called Survivors in Action (http://survivorsinaction.org). Very few people even know they exist. There is also the National Center for Victims of Crime, which operates the National Stalking Resource Center.

Survivors in Action points out that National Center does not operate a victim helpline, but offers fact sheets and brochures. The Stalking Resource Center asks for donations, but it appears those donations are mainly used to help fund conferences and trainings, as well as salaries.

The National Center for Victims of Crime does not specify in their IRS form 990 how much they receive in government grants (taxpayer funds) as they are not required to do so. The report does show they had total revenue of 3.5 million dollars and spent $156,000 on fundraising and two million for salaries, with other expenses adding up to nearly 1.5 million dollars.

If you go their website, you will find this notice for their Stalking Resource Center:

"*PLEASE NOTE: The National Crime Victim Helpline is closed. We regret the inconvenience. Please refer to our victim assistance resources. Are you being stalked (brochure-English and Spanish). Stalking Information. Stalking incident and Behavior Log."[37]

Survivors in Action says,

When a victim reaches the point where they need to call a Helpline, they need real help, not reading material . . . These are great tools, but where do victims actually turn to for help? . . . It can be assumed that funds are utilized for training that they provide to other organizations. . . but even their workshop/conferences range between $375–$575 to attend . . . It's hard to comprehend how they can manage to organize events but are unable to operate a helpline.

Survivors in Action posted this letter to the organization on their website that speaks directly to the issues:

There is nothing worse than being victimized by stalking and cyber stalking. I tried for months to get help. I reached out to any agency that I could locate including National Stalking Resource Center, National Crime Victims Bar, Domestic Violence agencies and law enforcement. No one would help me. I found Survivors In Action after watching an episode of Stalked Someone's Watching. SIA volunteers helped me create an events time line, taught me how to self-advocate and after only working with me for several days, I had support finally and was able to obtain a restraining order and get the local authorities to listen. There needs to be more agencies like

Survivors In Action that will provide direct support to stalking and cyber stalking victims. Thank you Alexis and SIA volunteers for all of your help. God Bless you all![38]

Rose S., Reno, NV

The Stalking Resource Center does provide training and conferences for local agencies, law enforcement, prosecutors, and other nonprofits and officials. So, it can be assumed that they do some good, even if not providing direct help for victims.

When we take a closer look at the type of conference they support, however, it is clear where the bias lies, and certainly these trainings are not going to pay any or very little attention to a significant number (as we have demonstrated in this chapter) of stalking victims: "The Stalking Resource Center, in partnership with the Battered Women's Justice Project and AEquitas: The Prosecutors' Resource on Violence Against Women, is excited to announce a national conference on Prosecuting Stalking Cases."[39]

Several webinars are also offered on "Prosecuting Stalking and Technology Cases" and "Intimate Partner Stalking," hosted by AEquitas, a resource for women—not for men.

Meanwhile, the National Network to End Domestic Violence (NNEDV) is the largest organization dealing with domestic violence, but in most areas, stalking victims are also referred to their associated organizations. This organization also does not provide any direct services to victims. They only provide information and training to the coalitions of service providers.

Survivors in Action opines:

Sue Else, President of the NNEDV states that programs around the country are *struggling* to provide life-saving services to victims (February 3, 2011) . . . *Is that really the reason for why many victims cannot get help? Are programs struggling?*. . . . Sue Else doesn't seem to be struggling at all, earning a six figure salary and benefits. As President, she has profited immensely in the last few years, bringing in nearly one million dollars in salary while her victims fund, Amy's Courage Fund, remains closed to victims due to a fund depletion because of 'high demand'. Fortunately, in 2009 Amy's Courage Fund helped 139 victims and $264,856 was paid out. In the same year, Sue made over $270,000—her salary totaling more than the entire victims fund. In 2008, Form 990 lists Sue Else's compensation as $267,870 and also lists the 'estimated amount of other compensation from the organization and other related organizations of $181,667, for a grand total of $449,537 . . . Clearly, money is not the issue, allocation and appropriation is.[40]

Is this feminism or FemMEism? Erin Pizzey is the founder of the battered women's movement since she opened the first shelter for abused women and wrote the first book on the subject, *Scream Quietly So the Neighbors Don't Hear*. She says of many of the women operating such shelters that are also supposed to help female stalking victims: "The activists aren't there to help women come to terms with what is happening in their lives. They're there to fund their budgets, their conferences, their traveling abroad, and their statements against men."[41]

Why is there no national hotline to help male and female stalking victims? Pizzey has provided the answer.

CHAPTER 4

Sexual Harassment

We begin with two personal accounts from correspondence to the author:

It was many years ago now, around 1990–91 I was a dishwasher at a (restaurant). Anyway it has always bothered me because all I ever hear about is Male on Female harassment and this time it clearly wasn't the case. At the time I was 18 and had just moved out. I was working hard and trying to get a job as a cook, as this would greatly help out with bills. Finally I got my chance. I would switch on and off as a dishwasher and cook taking time to learn the new job.

Well one day an assistant manager (Female) started to tell me what a good job I was doing. Telling me to keep up the good work, pats on the back and such. No harm there but then she started hanging out in the "dish pit" talking. Not a lot, but more than what a normal manager would do. Then one day she comes up behind me, real close and tells me in my ear "You're doing really good, here is a tip." Slipping a few bucks in my front pocket. Now to be honest at the time I was flattered I didn't say no but I wasn't encouraging her either. I had JUST got a new Girlfriend who was just the sort a young 18 year old boy wanted. And even though the female manager was attractive I was very loyal and did not take advantage of the advances. And you may think. Hey that isn't so bad. She comes on to you, you don't do anything. No harm no foul. And at the time I felt the same. Then a few weeks later, I'm finally a full time cook on the schedule. Time to make some dollars, it pretty much doubled my paycheck and that was good because

I really needed the income. Then it happened I went to check the schedule for the next week (they did them weekly) and bam! I was off the cook schedule and back to washing dishes. I go to the manager on duty that made the schedule and guess who it is . . . yep, her. I go to the office and I ask her what's up with the change. She tells me to step inside the office (very small I might add) she closes the door. I'm thinking wow I must have really messed up or something. But then she closes the blinds on the window and door. She starts with telling me that I was taken off the schedule because I was lacking. To which I replied. But you have been telling me I was doing great what's different now! She starts playing with papers on the desk with one hand while rocking the chair back and forth looking at me. Then she said something I'll never forget. "If you want back on the cook schedule . . . you have to show me. . . . show me how bad you want it." I just turned around and walked out I didn't even bother to quit. Turned in my work stuff and got my last check a week later.

Now looking back I know what I should have done, which was tell the general manager (also female), but I honestly didn't think anyone would believe me. I had zero proof. And even if I did I would have been laughed at. Something like a year or two later I stopped back in that (restaurant) to have a meal, see who was there, and talk to old friends, but almost everybody had moved on. Then I asked, "Hey is (manager's name) still here?" The server and busser began to chuckle I asked what was so funny? They said she wasn't there. She had gotten demoted and moved to another store. Apparently she got busted having sex with a cook in the walk freezer during her shift. I guess she was so loud you could hear it all the way from the back to the non-smoking section.

Maybe I should have said something told some one. I may have not been believed at the time. But after that craziness I would have. Looking back she was a single mom with a 60–70 hour a week job and wanted some sex but didn't have time to make a relationship. I was young and she knew I was in a position where I really needed the money. She probably figured I was safe, an easy mark. She was right I never told anybody.

Now I have a great job a loving wife and child it's probably for the best I didn't stay and give her what she wanted. My life was really changed by that decision I was unemployed for three months gained a bunch of weight, got depressed, and eventually drove my then girlfriend away. Because of all the crap that transpired after that decision I eventually pulled myself up and out, becoming an independent man who is beholden to no one. Please if you use any of this keep my email and name private.

One More Personal Account

The above story is about the experience of a young man just entering the workforce. Thank goodness, he was able to overcome the adversity he experienced at his first full-time job. He discusses the negative impact the sexual harassment had on him, which caused him to go into a depression. As stories were researched for this book, we continued to find instances where women were the aggressors in sexually fueled situations. Sexual harassment, however, does not necessarily occur between supervisors and subordinates at work, as the next account demonstrates:

Dear Mr. Cook:

I'm afraid my story itself doesn't sound too compelling. There were a lot of emotions that went into these series of events that are hard to describe in a few words. I wasn't groped or fired or the subject of some other tangible event. But that didn't make it any less painful.

I don't believe my specific story is the focal point. The real issues are: 1. The (lack of) response from my school; and 2. the personal aftermath.

The most telling aspect is the double standard I received (e.g., my "testing" by sending the letters and changing the genders). Whether it is domestic violence, harassment, or other problems, men are likely to be ignored. I used to think "justice will prevail," but not anymore.

The personal aftermath is that my experience caused me to pretty much shun a life in academics. I didn't want anything to do with the academic world nor did I want to associate with the same people or the same field of research. So I basically changed careers. In the end, it's worked out fine, but it does illustrate the impact.

This happened in 198_–198_ when I was a graduate student at . . . not harassment in the sense of employer-on-employee or professor-on-student harassment. It was student-on-student. The harassment itself may not very significant to you, although it was very significant to me at the time. But the real issue is how the situation was handled, or not handled, by my school.

A female student and I were working on the same general project. We were friends at the time. This was when we were both preparing for our PhD qualifying exams, which in my department were taken at about the one to half year mark of graduate school. As part of the exam process, we had to perform and defend two "mini" research projects.

At the time, the woman was having an affair with a married man. I really didn't understand this in the sense that she and the man (also a student) seemed like nice people. One thing else I noticed was that this woman often claimed that other men were in love with her (other students, professors, etc.). Again, I didn't really understand this but I accepted this at face value. I think she was having difficulty balancing the "workload" of the affair and her research projects. She performed little work on the project that I was associated with. More and more, I found myself helping her with this work. Better said, I was doing work for her. As an example, I would process data for her, and she would refer to it as "her work." In addition, she took computer codes from me and claimed them as her own. I had to get up at three in the morning and deliver needed field equipment to another school for her.

Needless to say, this and more created a lot of resentment on my part. This went on for perhaps 6 months to a year, spanning our qualifying exams.

I finally told her that she wasn't doing her share of the work and that I didn't like doing it for her. She didn't take this very well. A month before this she and her married boyfriend gave me a kitten for my birthday. The last thing in the world I needed was another living being to care for. I was spending huge amounts of time in my office, and didn't have time to physically or emotionally deal with a pet. Nor did I have any money. I didn't tell either of them that I didn't want a pet because I thought it would hurt their feelings. There was also the responsibility issue. The woman said, "Make sure you take him to the vet because they have a return policy at the pet store." I always thought that a person is supposed to care for an ill pet. Once again, a sign of a character flaw in her that I should have recognized. A sick animal needs help, not disposal. Well, the kitten was not eating and I did take him to the vet. It ended up costing me $1,500 that I didn't have. I didn't know if this little animal that depended entirely on me would live or die.

The most bizarre part of this was that both the woman and I lived in the same student housing complex. Pets were not allowed. But that didn't stop the woman from getting a dog a year earlier. The housing office found out, and gave her an eviction notice. So she gives me a cat. At the time, I assumed that the pet policy was being changed because no one who was being evicted from their own apartment for having a pet would give another person living at the same complex a pet. But I was wrong. I don't understand this to this day. I was evicted. It's even more bizarre but I'll leave that for another day.

I was struggling with my own work (and hers) at the time. The stress was unbearable. Add a sick pet to the mix. Add an eviction. I was suicidal at the time.

The harassment began after I told this woman that she was not doing her share of the work and that I didn't like doing her work for her, she was upset with me. From then on there was considerable animosity between us. For the next 6–12 months she began telling people that I was in love with her. In fact, she told people that I was suicidal because I was in love with her.

This may seem insignificant, but you have to be in my shoes. I'm struggling in graduate school. This woman takes credit for my work. She steals computer codes from me. She gives me a sick cat that I don't want or can't afford. Ultimately, this causes me to get evicted from my student apartment. Then she tells people that my feelings are caused by my being in love with her.

The spreading sexual stories/rumors about a person in the workforce are considered harassment. I was even more upset when I found out that this was happening. We did not get along well.

I tried to stop this woman from saying things about me that were not true. I went to faculty, the dean, the school vice president, human relations advisor, and I was ignored. I was told to "forget about it," "it's no big deal." I was even told that my complaints could jeopardize my chances of getting a degree. The human relations advisor—the person students were supposed to go to with issues such as this—was a radical feminist (I know that now). She was completely oblivious to my feelings. She rolled her eyes when I said I'd be treated differently if I was a woman.

After being ignored by the administration I knew what to do. I wrote anonymous letters to members of the staff and administration who were listed as ombudspeople for harassment and other complaints. The letters were sent through a woman friend. In six letters I stated my situation as it was (male harassed by female). I didn't receive a single response. In seven letters I reversed the genders (female harassed by male). Six of the seven responded back. All said I was harassed. They said they couldn't believe the treatment I received. Some suggested I seek legal action and sue. Boy, are things treated differently when it is a woman claiming harassment!

Twenty years later I graduated from ——— with a PhD. I left and never looked back. I had 13 job offers, including 2 faculty positions. I wanted nothing to do with the way men were treated in academia so I took a job at a . . . national laboratory. I've never been married. Why risk it? The odds are not good and family law does not favor men. Now at 50, I'm ready for early retirement. I have no regrets about my life.

My cat passed away five years ago after living for almost eighteen years. He provided me with a lot of love. I certainly wasn't wrong for taking responsibility for him over twenty years ago.

A Headline Story

Police Chief Accused of Sexually Assaulting Her Officers

A flurry of complaints and mounting grievances alleging sexual misconduct, illegal management practices and retaliation have been lodged against Paso Robles' first female chief of police, Lisa Solomon . . . The criticisms against Solomon include allegations of sexual assaults, many committed in the presence of others, repeated affairs with a list of subordinates, and bearing a child out of wedlock fathered by a former lieutenant in the department. . . .

In 2008, Solomon required all members of the command staff to attend a team-building workshop at the Carmel Valley Lodge during Super Bowl weekend. While there, Solomon allegedly sexually assaulted two officers, according to four officers who told CalCoastNews they were present at the time . . . Solomon . . . ordered the seven attending officers to the hot tub for a mandatory meeting. . . .

Shortly after they suited up and sat down in the tub, Solomon said, according to the men, "You wanna see boobs?" She removed her top and allegedly rubbed her breast in a commander's face, officers said. She then scooted up close to Sgt. Brennen Lux, slid her hand into his shorts and grabbed his penis. . . .

Solomon then reportedly turned her focus on Lt. Tim Murphy, whom she also groped. . . . City Manager Jim App declined to comment on the alleged investigation. He also demurred when asked why Solomon was not on administrative leave. . . .

Solomon was appointed chief of the 30,000-resident city in 2007. She was the first woman to hold positions of sergeant, lieutenant and captain in the department.

During her 20-year career in Paso Robles, she has been past president of the North County Women's Shelter and *chair of the San Luis Obispo County Sexual Assault Recovery and Prevention Program* (emphasis added).[1]

The next question we might want to ask is whether or not a man in Solomon's position would have immediately been put on administrative leave, pending investigation of such charges. A cursory internet search quickly found several examples in 2011:

Zachary, (Louisiana) The Attorney General's Office is investigating sexual harassment claims against the Assistant Police Chief of Zachary.

Darryl Lawrence is on paid administrative leave during the investigation.

Interim Police Chief David Courtney says the complaints came in last week and are from two female officers. He tells News 2 both claims against Lawrence are similar in nature. One involves direct contact, the other in-direct. News 2 learned the allegations are that Lawrence kissed one female officer, and sent sexually-explicit text messages to another.

Chief Courtney passed the investigation along to the AG's office, "because of the magnitude of the case."[2]

Mountainburg, (Arkansas) Mayor Ralph Bryant says Police Chief Barry Gudgeon is on unpaid administrative leave after several women filed sexual harassment complaints. Bryant confirms the city is conducting an internal investigation.

Bryant says he received four written and about a half dozen verbal sexual harassment complaints about Gudgeon. In a letter dated Sept. 6, 2011, the mayor tells Gudgeon citizens accused him of making "improper sexually related comments" while he was on duty and inside a patrol car.[3]

Then, there is this bizarre case from Concord, California, from 2012, which at least shows that those who sue sometimes are sued themselves:

> In what seems like a "she sued, she sued" soap opera, Concord agreed to settle with its employee Wendy Schwartzenberger, a civilian community service officer, for $150,000, which will be paid from city funds. According to the lawsuit that was filed last year, Lt. Robin Heinemann made unwelcome sexual remarks and physical advances, including patting Schwartzenberger's behind, hugging and kissing her "at least 100 times."
>
> In 2009, forty-six-year-old Heinemann, a 23-year department veteran and the highest-ranking woman in the Concord Police Department, filed a lawsuit against the city claiming that she was harassed and discriminated against because of her gender. Heinemann said she was the target of "trumped-up" internal-affairs investigations into whether she had been dishonest and disrespectful to superiors. According to the suit, male officers who were accused of wrongdoing went unpunished. Heinemann and her attorneys, Stan Casper and Toni Lisoni, settled with the city for $150,000.
>
> It doesn't stop there. More than a decade ago, Heinemann and other female police officers cried sexual harassment within the department and settled for $1.25 million. Heinemann was promoted to lieutenant two years later.[4]

In May 2012, at the West Midlands police department in England, things got even stranger:

> A lesbian police community support officer sexually assaulted five colleagues, fondling one woman's breasts and groping a male officer in his patrol car, a court heard yesterday.
>
> Sylvia Cooper, 45, subjected officers of both genders to a string of unwanted sexual advances, persistently touching their genitals and slapping their bottoms, it is alleged.
>
> On one occasion, she reached under a WPC's skirt from behind, while on another she grabbed a male officer while he was wearing cycling shorts and complimented him on his 'nice package', the court heard.
>
> Cooper is said to have treated the assaults 'as a joke' but officers were so uncomfortable they switched shifts to avoid contact with her.
>
> One female colleague requested a transfer because she was scared Cooper would touch her in the police station's changing rooms.

Cooper appeared in court yesterday accused of eight sexual assaults against colleagues at West Midlands Police when she worked as a PCSO in 2009 and 2010. She has been suspended from the force.[5]

What Is Sexual Harassment?

Some people do experience a "hostile work environment" that is detrimental to their efficiency and effectiveness on the job and it all has to do with sex. Sexually suggestive comments and inappropriate touching are two things that can affect the work climate and can negatively impact the victims and the company's bottom line. The term "Sexual Harassment" was coined in the 1960s with the passage of the Civil Rights Act of 1964. While the Civil Rights Act deals with a variety of discriminatory practices, Title VII deals specifically with the workplace environment. The law began to be implemented in 1965 and a number of cases have made national headlines. The law has had a widespread society-changing impact.

In 1979, feminist author Catharine MacKinnon published a book entitled *The Sexual Harassment of Working Women*, where she developed an argument that such harassment was a violation of civil rights. The Equal Employment Opportunity Commission (EEOC) expanded its definition of civil rights violations in the workplace to include sexual harassment in 1980. The first case that established the concept of a sexual harassment as a hostile working environment was *Meritor v Vinson* in 1986.

In 1988, a U.S. Court of Appeals found in *Hall v. Gus Construction* that even if conduct was not specifically sexual, when construction workers hazed female workers, it was gender-based harassment. In 1990, the EEOC decided that while isolated incidents of consensual favoritism do not violate the law, sexual advances that are unwelcome or widespread favoritism that becomes an unspoken condition of employment would be a violation of Title VII.

One of the most well-known American allegations of sexual harassment in the workplace is the scandal involving Supreme Court nominee Clarence Thomas and Anita Hill, which surfaced in October 1991. Thomas was the first African American nominated for the U.S. Supreme Court since Thurgood Marshall (1967) and was thought by many to be a great candidate. Anita Hill worked for Thomas at the U.S. Department of Education and later at the EEOC. She accused him of unwanted sexual advancements along with showing her some sexually explicit photos: "He spoke about acts that he had seen in pornographic films involving such matters as women having sex with animals and films showing group sex or rape scenes. . . . On several occasions, Thomas told me graphically of his own sexual prowess. . . . Thomas was drinking a Coke in his office, he got up from the table at which we were working, went over to his desk to get the Coke, looked at the can and asked, "Who has put pubic hair on my Coke?"[6]

Some senators questioned why Hill would follow Thomas to the EEOC from the Department of Education if he was sexually harassing her. Thomas was eventually confirmed by the U.S. Senate. Because the congressional hearings were televised, it made the general public more aware of sexual harassment in the workplace. That the hearings turned into a messy affair of "he said, she said" simply demonstrated the difficulty of such cases. Supporters of Hill had bumper stickers that said, "I believe her." Supporters of Thomas were quieter but doubtful of Hill's assertions.

The legal definition of sexual harassment describes the act as a form of sexual discrimination composed of three forms of behavior—quid pro quo harassment (this for that), "submission to or rejection of such conduct by an individual is used as the basis for employment decisions affecting such individual," and hostile work environment harassment.[7]

Different Standards for Men and Women

In 1991, in *Ellison v. Brady*, the Ninth Circuit Court of Appeals ruled that males and females could be treated differently when it comes to sexual harassment in the workplace. Instead of a reasonable person as a standard, such cases could be judged by a "reasonable woman" standard. The case involved a man's unsolicited love letters. The court decided that such letters and other unwanted attention might not seem inoffensive to the average man, but could be offensive to the average woman, and thus create a hostile work environment. As importantly, this ruling meant that court decisions could be based on what the complaining person believed to be harassment, not what the defendant thought or intended.

Another 1991 case, *Robinson v. Jacksonville Shipyard* found that when it comes to crude language, nude pin-ups or pornography in a locker room, and sexual graffiti, even if a specific person was not the target of such depictions, Title VII was a "sword to battle such conditions."[8] This important case established the principle that off-color or sexual jokes at the office were now subject to possible court action.

In 1993, the U.S. Supreme Court issued its second ruling regarding employment-based sexual harassment. In *Harris v. Forklift Systems*, the court found that even if an employee's psychological well-being is not affected, harassment exists if the employee subjectively perceives a hostile work environment and the conduct was severe and pervasive.

Later that same year, in *Burns v. McGregor Electronics Industries*, the 8th Circuit Court of Appeals ruled that even though a woman posed nude for magazines, it did not affect her claim that she found the workplace to be offensive.

In another (1996) case, in which male and female workplace conduct was judged differently, a federal district court in Kansas dismissed the discrimination suit of a male supervisor who was fired for participating in an office party in which a female subordinate was received as a birthday gift. In *Castleberry v. Boeing Company*, the court found that the male supervisor could be held to a higher standard (being fired as a consequence) while the female subordinate received only very mild disciplinary action.

A U.S. appeals court ruled (*Shepard v. Slater Steels Corporation*, 1999) that a male employee could sue due to vulgar language from a male co-worker, even if much of the conduct was not sexual, and the alleged victim was not gay. Importantly, this ruling helped further cement the concept that words and conduct of the alleged harasser must imply that they are motivated by gender.

The 7th Circuit Court of Appeals acted to further the distinction that sexual harassment to be actionable should be rooted in a gender bias. This case (*Holman v. Indiana*) revolved around a supervisor and a man and woman who were husband and wife. The supervisor solicited sex from both of them. The court ruled that an equal opportunity harasser did not discriminate because of gender, and therefore, there was no actionable claim. The 8th Circuit Court of Appeals agreed, by ruling against the plaintiff in a case involving foul language (*Hocevar v. Purdue Frederick Company*). The court found that such language was used in front of both men and women, so it was not a case of gender discrimination.

The High Court Takes Further Action

By 1998, the U.S. Supreme Court took up the issue three more times, ruling that men as well as women and same-sex cases can bring sexual harassment claims to court, and that even though there may not have been a tangible showing of loss of employment or promotion, a hostile work environment can exist, unless (for the first time, providing a more clear guideline for employers) the employer took reasonable care to correct and prevent such harassment and the employee took reasonable care to avoid harm. In other words, if an employee failed to use an established and clear complaint procedure, then the employer could avoid paying damages.

By 2004, the Supreme Court gave further clarification, ruling in *Pennsylvania State Police v. Suders* that employers have a valid defense if the complaining employee failed to use a reasonable system set up to report sexual harassment.

What the Data Shows

The U.S. EEOC keeps the statistical data on workplace sexual harassment claims, which is a federal offense. In 2008, the EEOC reported that 13,867 claims of sexual harassment were filed by employees against their employers. While we know the legal definition of sexual harassment, it is still a hard concept to define. Life experiences and perspectives shape the way people view social interactions. What may appear offensive to one person may be seen as funny to another; actions are open to interpretation and are subjective. Men and women perceive certain things differently. For example, men "typically haven't had a lifetime of experiences dealing with sexual harassment and may not know how to deal with it when it happens to them."[9] The number of men actually being sexual harassed in the workplace is probably substantially larger than what is reported, but because of perception, men may fail to perceive sexual remarks or touching as "inappropriate." When discussing sexual harassment, what comes to most people's mind is that of a woman being harassed by male colleagues, but what about men who are victims; can males be victims of sexual harassment? Out of the 13,867 document cases of sexual harassment in 2008, 15.9 percent were reported by men. Even though the statistics document sexual harassment cases happening to males, they do not divulge the gender of the assailant, but as more women are in positions of authority in the workforce, it stands to reason that the majority of the offenders against males are females. According to the study by the U.S. Merit Systems Protection Board,[10] 21 percent of men who report being harassed were harassed by other men. We can thus make the case that *about 80 percent of workplace harassment complaints by men are due to complaints about the actions of women.*

This chart does show the remarkable increase in male official complaints acted upon by the EEOC, from 1992 to 2001:

	1992	1993	1994	1995	1996	1997	1998	1999	2000	2001
Total charges:	10,532	11,908	14,420	15,549	15,342	15,889	15,618	15,222	15,836	15,475
Charges filed by men (%):	9.1	9.1	9.9	9.9	10.0	11.6	12.9	12.1	13.6	13.7[11]

As we shall see, more recent figures show an even greater increase than the 4.6 percent increase detailed in the chart from 1992–2001.

The percentage of male sexual harassment cases has doubled since 1990, from 8 percent to 16 percent in 2007.

Ernest Haffner, of the legal counsel's office at the EEOC acknowledges that they do not keep records of same-sex harassment. Haffner adds however, that the percentage and absolute numbers of complaints filed by men are higher than 10 years ago.

Even more telling, the *total* number of sexual harassment complaints by men and women has dropped over the same period. In 1997, 15,889 complaints were filed, compared with 12,510 in 2007.

Haffner points out that Supreme Court decisions, including one in 1998, laid out preventative measures employers could take to reduce the chance of being held liable in such situations, thus affecting the total number of complaints being filed.[12]

Memo from the Legal Department

Employment law attorney Mark Hammons says that, certainly, part of the reason for the increase is that more women are in management positions:

> Because you have more women in a position where they can act out, you will have an increased number of men who are victims of sexual harassment. When the management work force was almost exclusively male, you didn't see much of that, because there practically wasn't an opportunity for women to engage in the same bad behavior that men did . . . We've seen an increase in our practice on the number of men who are (not embarrassed as they once might have been) to complain. I think it's corrected a little bit more readily in the workplace when it comes from a co-worker, but there's still a lot of toleration of co-workers making sexual comments or comments that are demeaning. Men may come across the just get over it mentality that women used to encounter. There's still,

(however) probably more of that toward men, in making complaints.
I think there's probably a little bit more tendency to not take seriously a man's compliant or recognize that it may affect his work
environment as much.[13]

The U.S. EEOC recently made a surprising revelation showing that
sexual harassment complaints from men have risen by 16.4 percent
(2,094 claims) in 2010,[14] since the start of the recession.

Although almost totally focused as an organization on the physical
or sexual abuse of women, a report by the American Association of
University Women (AAUW), *Drawing the Line: Sexual Harassment on
Campus,* documents that women and men are equally likely (35% female to 29% male) to be sexually harassed on college campuses. Some
highlights from that report:

Most victims don't report sexual harassment. More than one-third
of college students do not tell anyone about their experiences with
sexual harassment. Those who do confide in someone usually tell
a friend. Female students are more likely to talk to someone about
their experiences than are male students, but less than 10 percent
of all students report incidents of sexual harassment to a college or
university employee. Students offer a range of reasons for why they
do not report incidents, including fear of embarrassment, guilt about
their own behavior, skepticism that anyone can or will help, and not
knowing whom to contact at the school. Still, the top reason that
students give for not reporting sexual harassment is that their experience was not serious or "not a big deal." Other than to say it is
unwanted sexual behavior, college students do not appear to have a
common standard for defining sexual harassment. Moreover, college
students are reluctant to talk about sexual harassment openly and
honestly and are more apt to joke or disregard the issue despite their
private concerns. This reticence to engage in a serious dialogue about
the issue may contribute to the prevalence of sexual harassment on
campus, as students interpret one another's silence as complicity. At
the very least it is an indication that college students don't have a
common understanding of where to draw the line. The ramifications
of sexual harassment can be serious. Sexual harassment can damage the emotional and academic well-being of students, provoke and
exacerbate conflict among students, and contribute to a hostile learning environment. For colleges and universities, sexual harassment can
be financially costly and damage their reputations. More broadly,

society as a whole is affected as graduating students bring their attitudes about sexual harassment into the workplace and beyond.[15]

A review of the academic literature shows that feminist theory dominates the discourse about sexual harassment. The vast majority of articles and studies done about sexual harassment in the workplace only examine women as victims, not as perpetrators.

The Independent Women's Forum featured an ad campaign on some colleges that sought to dispel what they considered "Feminist Myths." Here is what they said:

> Consider for example this statement: "Our schools are training grounds for sexual harassment . . . boys are rarely punished, while girls are taught that it is their role to tolerate this humiliating conduct." **Fact:** "Hostile Hallways," is the best-known study of harassment in grades 8–11. It was commissioned by the American Association of University Women (AAUW) in 1993, and is a favorite of many harassment experts. But this survey revealed that girls are doing almost as much harassing as the boys. According to the study, "85 percent of girls and 76 percent of boys surveyed say they have experienced unwanted and unwelcome sexual behavior that interferes with their lives." (Four scholars at the University of Michigan did a careful follow-up study of the AAUW data and concluded: "The majority of both genders (53%) described themselves as having been both victim and perpetrator of harassment— that is most students had been harassed and had harassed others." And these researchers draw the right conclusion: "Our results led us to question the simple perpetrator-victim model . . . ") (See: *American Education Research Journal*, Summer 1996).[16]

When men are victims, there seems to be disbelief that such a thing could happen to a man since our society is still understood to be patriarchal. A problem with gaining data about sexual harassment cases involving males is that the phenomena have been largely overlooked until recently. "Social science researchers like courts, are slow to take up forms of harassment that do not fit our top down, male-female sexual come on image of harassment."[17] Men can be victims of sexual harassment, as the EEOC statistical data documents. The U.S. EEOC recognizes that men have been victims of unwanted sexual attention; one of the sexual harassment guidelines states that "the victim as well as the harasser may be a woman or a man; the victim does not have to be of the opposite sex."[18]

One such case of heterosexual men harassing other men at work is the case of *Doe v. Belleville*. Older heterosexual men were found to have been harassing younger twin brothers at work for failing to be what the offenders claim "masculine enough in appearance and/or behavior."[19] One of the perpetrators even grabbed one of the twins by his genitals to confirm to the rest of the harassers that he indeed was male. The offenders created a hostile work environment by continuously teasing the twins and asking about their sexual orientation. The Seventh Circuit Court sided with Doe and agreed that they had legal rights guaranteed under Title VII of the Civil Rights Act of 1964 to not be harassed at work.

Types of Sexual Harassment

Sexual harassment can occur in a variety of circumstances, including but not limited to the following:

- The harasser can be the victim's supervisor, an agent of the employer, a supervisor in another area, a co-worker, or a non-employee.
- The victim does not have to be the person harassed but could be anyone affected by the offensive conduct.
- Unlawful sexual harassment may occur without economic injury to or discharge of the victim.
- The harasser's conduct must be unwelcome.[20]

Sexual harassment continues to hamper employment opportunities for many men and women.[21] The EEOC and Fair Employment Practice Agencies document that sexual harassment claims filed by men in the U.S. workforce rose in 1998, 2000–2002, 2004, 2006–2007, and 2009.[22] Men being sexually harassed at work is a newly documented phenomenon that has been underexplored by scholars and the media. The whole concept of a man being the victim of sexual harassment was relatively unheard of until recently, in part because of our ideology of men as the stronger gender, the protector of society. One study of government employees, however, found that out of 8,000 surveys returned that questioned experiences of sexual harassment in the workplace, 19 percent of male respondents had experienced it within the previous two years.[23]

The First Court Case Is Followed by Increased Complaint Rates

The first case of a male (Mr. Papa) alleging sexual harassment by a female boss was brought against Domino's Pizza by the federal government and heard in the Federal District Court in Tampa in 1995. It was substantiated that his female boss had touched and squeezed his buttocks on numerous occasions. When Mr. Papa responded by expressing his frustration of the unwelcomed sexual advances to his boss, the offender, she fired him one week later, disguised as a problem with some accounting issues.[24]

In 2009, Regal Entertainment agreed to pay a male employee $175,000 because a sexually hostile work environment was created due to sexual harassment he received from a female colleague. The female colleague was accused of continuously grabbing the male employee's crotch. When the victim, along with his immediate supervisor, complained to the general manager, she retaliated by giving the victim low work performance evaluations. EEOC documents that sexual harassment charges filled by men have increased over the past decade from 12 percent to 16 percent. David Grinberg, a spokesman for the EEOC stated that "sexual harassment filings by men have consistently increased, doubling over 15 years."[25] EEOC attorney Mary Jo O'Neill says that for male harassment victims, "everyone expects that they would be able to handle it and take care of it themselves."[26] Might this expectation be especially strong if the harasser is a member of "the weaker sex?"[27] A study conducted by Street et al. on military reservists' shows that men and women who are victims of sexual harassment have been associated with more negative mental health issues.[28] Hall claims that sexual harassment is linked to anxiety, stress, and depression.[29] Street et al. advocate for clinicians to increase their awareness of the potential of sexual harassment happening to men, in order to provide the male victims with the appropriate care. Some of the consequences of being a victim of sexual harassment at work, noted by Hall (1994), are low job satisfaction and high absenteeism.[30]

As women have become increasingly prominent in the workforce with greater positions of power and authority in supervisory and management positions, we can expect a continued increase in the extent, nature, and consequences of sexual harassment in the workplace that are directed against male co-workers.

Another Memo from the Legal Department

The Naverette law firm in San Francisco has some advice for employers in this regard:

> In many cases, a manager or supervisor's first response to complaints of sexual harassment from a male employee is dismissal.

To be fair, in a majority of sexual harassment cases, the victim will be female. However, this is simply the norm and it's important to remember that anyone can become a victim of sexual harassment.

In a recent case, reported on by James L. Jorgensen at nwi.com, a man was repeatedly approached by a married female coworker. Despite complaints to four separate managers, nothing was done and the woman continued to make uninvited sexual overtures.

Finally, exasperated and out of supervisors to go to, the man sued the company, claiming they had allowed the prolongation of a hostile work environment. The company's excuse was that 'most men in the male employee's circumstances would have welcomed the (female coworker's) behavior.'

Flip that sentiment around.

Suppose that an employer defended a male employee's sexual advances or solicitation by saying that most female workers would have welcomed the attention. Most would find this grossly dismissive and offensive . . . For employers, if a male employee has complaints of sexual harassment, you have a duty to listen and, if appropriate, pursue corrective action.[31]

Training Bias?

The extent to which the advice of the legal profession is being followed by business and corporate firms is a matter for some speculation. The authors find that there are hundreds, if not thousands, of private and public professional speakers/trainers who specialize in presentations on the subject for businesses or as an aspect of business consulting and training. Certainly, there are many firms that seek to emphasize the need for their services, such as Alliance Training and Consulting: "Recent Supreme Court decisions, EEOC Guidelines, and many state laws . . . make it clear that employers need to go beyond simply having an anti-harassment policy. Employers need to ensure that management and supervisor harassment training is provided. Employers will also want to provide training to ensure every employee understands the organization's harassment policy."[32]

It is speculation however, given the sheer number of such firms, to assume that the issues of male harassment are either not addressed at all or given little emphasis in the majority of such presentations. A Google search result found confirmation for the top listed firm under "Sexual harassment in the workplace speaker's trainers."

The National Association of Working Women offered: "Learn how 9to5 trainers can help your firm or organization value and profit from diversity and enact effective policies and procedures to prevent sexual harassment."[33] Diversity Builder offered such training but seems to be primarily focused on African American and Gay Lesbian Bi Transgendered (LGBT) issues.[34] By the time we reached the third on the search list, that led us to other services that were more professional, and although a brief overview is all that we offer here, most of such trainings appear to be gender inclusive, with a good bit of awareness that there are many types of sexual harassment in the workplace with same gender and opposite gender instances as well as heterosexual male versus heterosexual woman, and yes, an acknowledgement that the reverse is possible as well in a heterosexual situation. There is no doubt, however, that despite an effort to be gender-inclusive in such trainings, it is clear that some offer only a one-gender perspective; and others lack balance.

The Real World of Work

Nevertheless, it would not be wildly speculative to assume that cultural norms are at not at play in the work arena as well.

We recall here an account in Warren Farrell's landmark book *The Myth of Male Power:*[35]

> Guy wrote to me that he had taken a picture of a woman at work who was sitting seductively in a miniskirt with her blouse unbuttoned enough to expose her bra (and some breast). He pinned the picture up on a file cabinet. The woman's face was turned away so she wasn't immediately recognizable.
>
> Guy's boss immediately called him into his office and ordered him to "remove the pornography from the file cabinet." When Guy explained, tongue-in-cheek, that it was "just a real-life picture of our work environment," the boss caught the joke and laughed, but still ordered him to remove the picture. **The woman however, whose picture was the "pornography," was not asked to dress in a less pornographic manner.** The workplace reality created by some females is, when photographed, the workplace pornography protested by other females.
>
> Months later, Guy was called in to the office again. His boss told him he was being fired from work because of complaints that he was "too interested in men's issues." None of these complaints documented any interference with his otherwise exemplary work

history. And Guy worked in a "male-dominated" profession under a male boss.

Guy's workplace porn was not expected to get the woman sexually turned on, yet Guy was fired despite the fact that a purpose of female flirtatious dress is to sexually activate men like Guy. Workplace porn (the male style that bothers only some females) is condemned while flirtatious dress (the female style that actively disturbs the great majority of the males) is protected.

Farrell's highly recommended book was the first to discuss the issue of workplace sexual harassment in a male inclusive manner, but it came out in 1993.

Has the picture changed since then? Would today's work climate be more likely to respond differently to a male complaint regarding female dress? No amount of investigation would reveal a definitive answer, but our sense is that things have changed to some extent. More government agencies and corporations have followed the high school example and instituted formal dress codes, stimulated by fear of sexual harassment complaints.

Men in general, and the data trend of complaints via the EEOC points this out, seem to be more likely to respond in a more previously perceived female-only fashion to workplace instances of sexual harassment.

Is Something Wrong with the Law?

Farrell and other authors find fault with the entire concept of sexual harassment in the workplace: "All forms of sexual contact at work and at school are best dealt with by the institution's improving communication rather than the government mandating legislation. . . . This is not a perfect solution. It is only more perfect than having government legislation of sexual nuance with its potential for annihilating anyone we dislike via a false accusation."[36]

He correctly points out that many marriages still take place because the romance started at a work-place that the two people shared: "Overall 35 million Americans report some kind of 'social-sexual' experience on their jobs each week. More than 80 percent of all workers say they've had such and experience on their job. When it works, we call it a wedding and the woman's picture is in the paper; when it doesn't, we call it a lawsuit and the man's picture is in the paper."[37]

In the 1998 book, *Heterophobia: Sexual Harassment and the Future of Feminism*, Professor Daphne Patai declares in the Preface that: "Except for egregious offenses such as assault, bribery or extortion (whether sexual or not)—for which legal remedies have been in place for many years—the petty annoyance of misplaced sexual attention or sexual put-downs has to be tolerated. Why? Because the type of vigilance necessary to inhibit it would create a social climate so unpleasant and ultimately so repressive, that the cure would be much worse than the disease."[38]

Patai says such a social climate has been created with disastrous consequences for everyone. Wendy McElroy is a libertarian commentator and runs ifeminist.com. A supporter of Patai, in a speech delivered in 2002, she says that the underlying assumptions of sexual harassment policies and laws need to be challenged:

> First, that sexual harassment is based on assumptions that are not just anti-male, they are anti-female. Sexual harassment laws assume that women are not able to compete successfully with men on an even playing field, in a rough-and-tumble world of free speech: we are so weak and psychologically fragile as to require government protection in our social and professional interaction.
>
> I don't know about other women, but I refuse to have those words describe *me*. It is an insult . . . an insult to women that government has institutionalized into law.
>
> Second, it is important to hammer in the toll of human misery that has been inflicted upon those who are accused of sexual harassment. At universities, those accused have no presumption of innocence . . . that is something they must prove to committees that often has the power to ruin their lives. They have no right to face their accuser or to question witnesses, no right to a lawyer or even, necessarily, to know the exact charges being brought against them. And the charges can be brought for nothing more than assigning the wrong homework, telling the wrong joke, asking female students tough questions or not asking them enough questions.
>
> Daphne Patai is very good at driving home the savagery of sexual harassment laws and policies. One third of her book, part II, is entitled 'Typifying Tales.' There she offers real life stories. For example . . . one case . . . a very over-weight and by all accounts a very popular, competent professor responded to a taunt shouted out in class by a female student. She rudely commented on the extreme 'size' of his chest: in response, he observed that she had no such problem. A witch-hunt of sexual harassment charges ensued. It was so extreme that the professor committed suicide. In a press release, the university's main concern was that the professor's

death would not discourage other similarly "abused" women from "speaking out."

The abomination known as the sexual harassment industry must be swept away.[39]

Patai further argues that the main objective of Catharine MacKinnon and other radical feminists is the "dismantling of heterosexuality," but unable to directly achieve this objective, they have contrived an "obstacle course in the relations of men and women."[40] She argues that the mere allegation of sexual harassment gives women an extraordinary weapon that is traditional in some respects, but is now backed up in laws and regulations. She contends that the aim of such laws is to "bring men to heel."

Ellen Frankel Paul is professor of political science and deputy director of the Social Philosophy and Policy Center at Bowling Green State University in Bowling Green, Ohio. She contends in her article in *Society*, "Bared Buttocks and Federal Cases," that there needs to be a distinction between offensive behavior and behavior that causes harm. Behavior that may be morally offensive should not be matter for the law, while behavior that causes harm should be:

Do we really want legislators and judges delving into our most intimate private lives, deciding when a look is a leer, and when a leer is a Civil Rights Act offense? . . . Should people have a legally enforceable right not to be offended by others? At some point, the price for such protection is the loss of both liberty and privacy rights. . . .

Workplaces are breeding grounds of envy, personal grudges, infatuation, and jilted loves, No one, female or male, can expect to enjoy a working environment that is perfectly stress-free, or to be treated always and by everyone with kindness and respect. To the extent that sympathetic judges have encouraged women to seek monetary compensation for slights and annoyances, they have not done them a great service . . . Women cannot expect to have it both ways: equality where convenient, but special dispensations when the going gets rough. Equality has its price and that price may include unwelcome sexual advances, irritating and even intimidating sexual jests, and lewd and obnoxious colleagues.

Egregious acts—sexual harassment per se—must be legally redressable. Lesser but not trivial offenses, whether at the workplace or in other more social settings, should be considered moral lapses for which the offending party receives opprobrium, disciplinary warnings, or penalties, depending on the setting and the severity. Trivial offenses . . . unless they become outrageous through persistence or content, these too should be taken as part of life's annoyances . . . As the presence of women on road gangs, construction crews, and oil rigs becomes a fact of life, the animosities and tensions of this transition period are likely to abate gradually. Meanwhile, women should "lighten up," and even dispense a few risqué barbs of their own, a sure way of taking the fun out of it for offensive male boors.[41]

In her book, *What to Do When You Don't Want to Call the Cops: A Non-Adversarial Approach to Sexual Harassment*, and in subsequent articles, Joan Kennedy Taylor also decries the development of sexual harassment law and the majority of specialists who advise business and governments:

We are letting something destructive happen to American business in the name of helping women. Current sexual harassment law—that is, the extension of anti-discrimination law to stifle and punish sexual speech in the workplace—is creating the very hostility between the sexes that it purports to correct. Men and women are not natural enemies but are being told that they are. Men are warned that if they offend female co-workers they might be disciplined or even terminated. Women are being instructed that offensive speech, if heard from men in the workplace, is probably illegal. And to top it off, the Supreme Court is requiring businesses to give these warnings. There is certainly a free speech issue involved, but from a management perspective the matter is worse than that: it's divisive . . . Once more, an attempt to protect women at work is doing them harm. Like the labor legislation, sexual harassment protection spreads the assumption that women are too delicate to flourish in the workplace without government aid. Sexual harassment regulation has failed women in a changing world. It harms everyone. It violates free speech, creates rather than lessens workplace hostility and fosters a Victorian view of women. If some women find it difficult to speak up for themselves, we should help them empower themselves, not rely on the government to mandate worker relations.

Not only should government not be relied on in social situations, it cannot be relied on. Women can learn what to expect in the workplace and how to handle problems that arise with their male

co-workers. In so doing women will not only better protect themselves, they will also feel the satisfaction that comes from being
effective personally as well as professionally.[42]

Legal and economic scholars such as Kaushik Basu argue that there are
other problems as well:

> I shall argue that this tying up of sexual harassment with sex dis-
> crimination, though it has played an important role historically, is
> now becoming a hindrance. There should be strong laws to pre-
> vent discrimination and strong laws to prevent harassment. But it
> would be unfortunate if the only way to establish sexual harass-
> ment is to categorize it as a form of discrimination, because this
> approach raises a number of problems . . . Employment discrimi-
> nation by sex has traditionally meant men discriminating against
> women . . . But sexual harassment is a more complex topic. First,
> men's claims of sexual harassment are increasing . . . The coupling
> of sexual harassment with sex discrimination does not work neatly
> to protect people in such cases.
>
> Second, in the United States, there is a significant amount of
> same-sex harassment, another situation in which law based on
> discrimination according to sex often does not provide adequate
> protection to sufferers—and when it does, it is only because judges
> and lawyers interpret the law according to its likely intent rather
> than what it actually says. . . . A third category that is difficult
> within the sex discrimination framework involves the problem of
> the boss who harasses both men and women with equal vigor and
> thus does not harass anybody because of his or her sex . . . A final
> category is those who are harassed not because of their sex, but
> because of their sexual orientation.[43]

An argument can also be made that there exists a more litigious society in general, and that such suits consume an inordinate amount of
resources and help to stifle economic growth.

An Uncomfortable Fact

Men face sexual harassment by women in the workplace and in other
life arenas, but it is an uncomfortable fact. That women face the same
kinds of issues is also a fact, but not so uncomfortable to accept and
act upon. This is demonstrated mainly by personal accounts of which

we have offered only a few examples here. The consequences for men experiencing these events are similar to those that women experience. From a business perspective, there is a demonstrable loss in productivity, and possible loss of a valued employee. There are obvious losses too for the affected man, emotionally, financially, in family life as well as the potential for being falsely accused. The potential for a false allegation of sexual harassment is still more likely even, given today's cultural norms to occur to a man than a woman. This as well, must be considered for what it is—sexual harassment—which is a form of sexual abuse.

A Middle Ground?

Our purpose here is not to examine sexual harassment law in detail, nor propose remedies. That is best left to other authors who have done so, or will do so. It deserves full-length treatment as a single subject. Rather, we wish to simply examine whether or not sexual harassment also affects a significant number of men, examine some of the consequences of those instances, and look at whether such incidents are similar or dissimilar from the experiences of women.

It is regrettable that teachers can no longer talk privately to students, that friendly hugs between the sexes are banned, that sexual banter of the most innocuous sort is subject to condemnation with possible adverse legal or career consequences; and that lives have been and are being destroyed by those less interested in the redress of legitimate grievances than by power and control. We have some further examples of this in the final chapter.

Somewhere out there are a man and his wife and his two children perhaps teaching in a high school or junior college. He certainly is no longer a college professor. I don't think I've ever met a more confused and more befuddled man and wife. They came to a workshop on gender issues to try and understand what had happened to them.

He was a college professor teaching history, and gave a star student of the women's studies department a failing grade. He met with her several times (with the door to his office open) in an attempt to get her to do additional work to bring the grade up. This attempt was unsuccessful. She later went to the head of her department and complained that in his talks with her, she felt like she was "verbally raped."

He was not given the tenure he had been expecting and eventually left with little hope of getting hired at another university.

I had some analysis for him and his wife as to why this happened to him, and how it could occur. Such analysis provided little solace.

It does seem however, that Joan Kennedy Taylor and others can point us in the right direction.

Increased communication and gender-inclusive training in how to achieve it seems to be a better way to go in the workplace than litigation or other forms of punishment. The consequences for making false charges should be as severe as the consequences for the alleged harassment.

Finally, to achieve some balance, we perhaps as a society need to include in our lexicon of sensitivity training an element of *de-sensitizing training*. We began this chapter with two stories from men. The first was a clear-cut case of quid pro quo—accede to sexual demands or risk losing a job as was the third headline case allegedly involving the California female police chief. The second case involved the spreading sexual stories/rumors about a person in the workforce from a co-worker. He considered this harassment but was most upset about the double-standard he experienced (even going so far as to write complaint letters under a different gender name) and getting agreement that, if he was a woman, it would be considered harassment. Nevertheless, the quid pro quo type of incident or very intimidating sexual remarks and certainly physical acts are vastly different than spreading rumors or the occasional inappropriate remark or joke and should be treated as such both in the workplace reactions of supervisors, the legal sphere, and yes, even in the response of those experiencing such events.

It is not the purpose of this volume in any of the areas we shall discuss to compare data and demonstrate that men experience these events to a greater extent than women. It is useful to counter gross exaggerations of the data such as the mainly anti-gender-feminist politically conservative/libertarian groups like the Independent Women's Forum or other commentators have done, but its usefulness is limited to just that. Where the data clearly indicates that is the case (such as cyber stalking or false allegations, for example), we will highlight it. Regarding the subject of this chapter, suffice it to say that there are likely few women on the planet who have not been subjected to some sort of sexual harassment in their lives from the wolf whistle, the leer, the prolonged peer down the blouse, the off-color joke, the inappropriate remark, and so on. We must recognize and applaud the greater empowerment of women to confront such behavior when they find it objectionable and most especially when it interferes with workplace activities. That men are also feeling more empowered in a sense of being bolder in requesting equality in dealing with these matters is evident in the increase in EEOC filings. The "style" of conduct that may be sexual harassment and the other issues explored here, may be different in many cases when a woman does it to a man. The personal consequences of such conduct and his reaction to it may be similar in many respects, but there are as we have discovered, great differences, and those differences relate not so much to the incidents themselves, but the reaction of others.

CHAPTER 5

Considering the Unthinkable:
The Last Taboo

The Missing Part

We will start this chapter with a paragraph we intentionally deleted in the chapter on sexual harassment. It is from the second of our two lead-off personal stories. This was from the man who left academia after a sexual harassment episode with another student: "It was at that time that I became interested in men's rights. (I read your book *Abused Men: The Hidden Side of Domestic Violence* many years ago, I believe immediately after it was published—great book). I now know that the treatment of men is obscene in our society. Whether it's the press, culture, or laws; men are at a significant disadvantage. And when men seek help, they are most often ignored."

It is, unfortunately, an often hurled epithet that the progenitor of human rights is simply a promulgator of special rights for some. One is reminded again of Schopenhauer's dictum that any truthful idea goes through three stages—that of being ignored, that of being violently objected to, and then finally received as conventional wisdom.

What we have been examining here is simply what we hope is "interesting research into human behavior that has long been ignored."[1] and it is worth it in that regard alone. To link it to a "men's rights" movement, whatever one may wish that to be, is to reduce the majority of human interactions to the particulars of one gender, and then it is an unfortunate and easy leap to cast those same interactions also in terms of race, creed, sexual orientation, political affiliation, and so on. It then becomes, as Louis Menand so aptly opined in the *New Yorker*, in an article called the "War of All Against All"[2] where individual motives are ascribed to groups, and he noted as an example, that women are not more or less moral than men. They are simply part of a group, and that while one can benefit from association with others in a group, "Groups are essentially imaginary. Souls are real, and they can be lost or saved only one at time."

When I have spoken to college students (I do not get asked very often to speak on college campuses), I do ask them a series of questions and ask them to raise their hands. When you exclude any romantic or potentially romantic situations, which do you get along with best? This includes everyone you come in contact with in terms of friendliness and communication. Here are the choices:

Who do you get along with best?

A. I get along best with people of the same sex as me.
B. I get along best with people of the opposite sex than me.
C. It does not really matter what the sex of the other person is.

I do not have any idea what a true scientific survey would do with such a questionnaire, but it should be obvious to most reading this, that the overwhelming majority raise their hands to choose option C. About 10 percent of the students raise their hands and say they communicate better with either the same sex or opposite sex.

We also choose option C. That is, people should be and can be treated equally, based on who they are first and foremost. The results of our second letter writer's survey of university official's response to his harassment complaint when the genders were reversed are worth exploring. If there was evidence to support this kind of double standard being an isolated incident, it would be one thing, but common sense as well as the scientific evidence must inevitably point us to a different conclusion.

Gender Disparity

We will intentionally neglect, for the most part, a discussion of media images and whether or not men or women suffer more as a result in the popular culture of movies, television, the internet, comic strips, and popular song. It is an interesting subject of discussion certainly, but whether such popular depictions of the sexes and the sexual peccadillos or even sexual assaults of either are depicted more unfairly toward one sex versus the other seems to serve no purpose here. Besides, popular culture is a moving target that is best aimed at in the instant access of the internet.

We are, however, greatly interested in how government, and non-governmental agencies, corporations, groups, and helping professionals engage in gender discrimination. In particular, we are of course interested in how such policies and procedures impact services for what the best available evidence proves to be an underserved significant segment of the population.

The missing part is men. In an *Oregonian* editorial, I called men "A National Afterthought."[3] Pointing out that there are seven official government agencies dealing specifically with women, health, violence, and labor, for example; but none for men. There is a White House Council for Women and Girls but no council for men and boys. (Full disclosure here, I serve as a volunteer on a commission headed by Warren Farrell attempting to get the White House to create a council for men and boys. As of this writing, it has not been created, despite a request from the White House to Dr. Farrell to submit such a proposal.) Nearly every state has a commission for women, but only one—New Hampshire— has one for men as well.

There is also the federal Violence Against Women Act, even though more men suffer violence of all sorts than do women, and the fact that the domestic violence rate is equal or nearly equal for men and women. Efforts to change the name seem to have picked up steam a bit and it is now a bit of debate where 10 years ago, there was none at all. The argument for the naming of this act is that since the majority of the victims of domestic and sexual violence are women, it should be named for the majority of such victims. By this logic, of course, we should re-name the Occupational Safety and Health Administration to the *Men's* Occupational Safety and Health Administration because 90 percent of workplace injuries happen to men instead of women. This is so because among the top five most hazardous jobs—firefighting, logging, heavy trucking, construction, and coal mining—the jobs are 97–99 percent male. A number of other very hazardous occupations, such as commercial fishing for example, are almost exclusively male. The safest occupations, secretary and receptionist, for example, are 97–99 percent female. Almost as many men are killed at work each day as were killed during the average day in the war in Vietnam,[4] and much more than have been killed in Iraq and Afghanistan.

I found myself speaking privately recently with the Chief of Staff to a U.S. senator. The reason for the meeting was to talk about the gender disparity in government agencies. Why seven agencies for women and none for men? Could not the men at least have a department of men's health, for example? (Would not such a department then have some focus on sexual crimes against men as part of men's health?) He did not answer the question directly, but he asked, "How would you answer the position that the government is simply making up for the past when the needs of women were neglected?"

My answer was not very coherent at the time, but it is a fair question. One could come up with some possible pithy answers.

1. That is true, there was discrimination in the past against women, but hasn't the pendulum swung too far?
2. Shouldn't all people be treated equally? Why should one gender or sexual orientation, these days, be denied the same services given to another?

I do not think, however, that these answers are exactly the right one, but I did pass by Arlington Cemetery later that day, with the rows on rows of grave markers of those who have died in military service—many who were subject to the draft while women still do not even have to register with the Selective Service. The Defense Department recently made a change in policy to allow women in combat, which may enhance a legal challenge to this aspect of sexual discrimination. The penalty for 18-year-old men who fail to register for the draft is up to five years in jail and/or a fine of up to $250,000. Perhaps the answer should have been: "Well, which woman do you want to shoot first to make up for past discrimination?"

In any case, my appeal fell on deaf ears at the senator's office. Perhaps this was due to my lack of deftness of discussion on my part, a lack of apparent political clout, or any number of other reasons.

His response to the issues, however, is simply indicative of a current political culture that sees all programs and policies that benefit women in particular as good, while anything that is for men solely or even in part is seen as not worthy of attention.

This political overlay directly impacts the male as a victim of sexual abuse and their concerned friends and family in a directly verifiable way.

Lip Service

We draw the subtitle here from the excellent Kate Fillion book of the same title. It is a complete and thorough examination of how some groups, by and large for women, pay lip service to equality for all, but do not actually deliver on their public pronouncements. In terms of delivery for male victims of domestic violence, the case is well proven in a previous volume that discrimination, both overt and covert, exists against a substantial number of male victims of domestic abuse.

When it comes to male victims of sexual abuse, it is even worse. We simply have to come to the conclusion even based on the limited data available, that this segment of our population is woefully underserved, unacknowledged, discriminated against, laughed at, demeaned, and diminished. It is, however, a much larger population than most of us would think exists. Even contemplating the serious existence of such a population of heterosexual men, as Dr. George terms it, is the *last taboo*.

Researcher Cindy Struckman-Johnson puts it rather succinctly: "Our society has no place for the male victim of sexual assault" and that "Our culture's ignorance of male rape is compounded by the fact that most male victims do not report their experience to the police, health officials, or even to friends and family."[5]

Implications

The impact of this neglect on the victims themselves is what we would expect, for female victims under the same sets of circumstances, as we have explored in the research results reported in previous chapters. There may be as well a heightened and sometimes lifelong distrust of the other gender. The most serious events likely result in more serious consequences, such as suicide, substance abuse, divorce, increased physical and mental health problems, legal problems and more. The fiscal and psychic cost is borne by all of society, one way or the other.

Further Forms of Sexual Abuse of Adult Men by Adult Women

We have focused on four main types of such abuse—harassment, coercion and assault, stalking, and rape. There are others that should be considered as worthy of consideration within this category. For example, what about false allegations? Are these more often leveled at men rather than women? Are the accusations of abuse, either sexual or physical, more readily believed and acted upon by authorities? Should not false allegations also be considered and condemned as sexual abuse?

False Allegations as a Type of Abuse

First, we need to deal with some full disclosure by the author and then deal with the available facts. I served as a member of the board of directors for Stop Abusive and Violent Environments (SAVE) and the website is www.saveservices.org. I am no longer associated in any way with this organization. Other than the proposal for a White House Council for

Boys and Men, www.whitehouseboysmen.org, I have no active member-
ship in any other organization, although I do volunteer for Stop Abuse
For Everyone (www.stopabuseforeveryone.org). It is important here to
make a full disclosure of current and prior affiliations because one of the
purposes of SAVE has been to answer questions about false allegations of
abuse. I am cognizant of the limited research efforts of that group so far,
and they cannot answer very many questions about the extent, nature,
and consequences of false allegations—yet.

SAVE did pay, however, for what is apparently the first national survey regarding false allegations. Unfortunately, a scientific, nationally
represented-for-population type of poll was not affordable. It is what is
known as a random poll, but with enough general respondents to give
it some validity.

This was a national survey of 10,000 households and found that 11
percent of respondents stated they had been falsely accused of domestic
violence, child abuse, or sexual assault.[6]

A number of other studies however, have also looked at the percentage of abuse allegations that are false.

For example:

- The Canadian Incidence Study of Reported Child Abuse and Neglect analyzed data from 7,672 child maltreatment investigations.
  Among the 798 cases of alleged sexual abuse, only 38 percent were
  substantiated.[7]
- A major study in a Midwestern city over the course of nine years
  found 41 percent of all rape claims were false[8]
- An analysis of police records at two large state universities found 50 percent of the rapes reported to campus police were determined to be false.[9]
- An Air Force study evaluated 556 rape allegations, and concluded
  that *60 percent were false.*[10]

As part of the Air Force study, women who were found to have made
false accusations were asked, "Why?"

Motivations given by the women who acknowledged they had made
false accusations of rape:

Spite or Revenge—20%
To compensate for feelings of guilt or shame—20%
Thought she might be pregnant—13%
To conceal an affair—12%

To test husband's love—9%
Mental/emotional disorder—9%
To avoid personal responsibility—4%
Failure to pay, or extortion—4%
Thought she might have caught VD—3%
Other—6%

The study found that most false accusations are "instrumental"—they serve a purpose. If the purpose is not avoiding guilt or getting revenge, it might serve a more focused purpose, for example, telling her parents "I didn't just go out and get pregnant—I was raped"; or telling her husband, "I didn't have an affair; it wasn't my fault, I was raped."

- Since 1989, more than 250 persons convicted of rape have been exonerated and freed as a result of post-conviction DNA testing.[11]

In a report for the National Center for the Prosecution of Violence Against Women, the authors conclude: "Of course, in reality, no one knows—and in fact, no one can possibly know—exactly how many sexual assault reports are false. However, estimates narrow to the range of 2–8% when they are based on more rigorous research of case classifications using specific criteria and incorporating various protections of the reliability and validity of the research."[12]

Do we know with some degree of certainty how many people (male and female) are falsely convicted of all types of crime? Samuel R. Gross in a research paper for the University of Michigan School of Law succinctly sums up the state of our knowledge:

> How many are there? The answer, unfortunately, is almost always the same and always disappointing: We don't know. Recently, however, we have learned enough to be able to qualify our ignorance in two important respects. We can put a lower bound on the frequency of false convictions among death sentences in the United States since 1973, and we have some early indications of the rate of false convictions for rape in Virginia in the 1970s and early 1980s. These new sources of information suggest—tentatively—that the rate of false convictions for serious violent felonies in the United States may be somewhere in the range from 1% to 5%. Beyond that—for less serious crimes and for other countries—our ignorance is untouched.

Gross adds that the false rape conviction rate in which physical evidence was examined by the Virginia Department of Forensic Science from 1973 through 1987 found an innocent rate of least 3.2 to 5 percent, and "almost certainly quite a few more." He cautions, however, that this Virginia case study, important as it is, may not be representative of all rape cases in the United States. Speaking of all erroneous convictions in the United States, Gross asks some questions:

> Is that a lot or a little? That depends on your point of view. If as few as 1% of serious felony convictions are erroneous, that means that perhaps ten- to twenty-thousand or more of the nearly 2.3 million inmates in American prisons and jails (Glaze, 2011) are innocent, and thousands of new innocent defendants are locked up each year. If the rate is higher, these numbers will go up. If as few as 1/10 of 1% of jetliners crashed on takeoff, we would shut down every airline in the country. That is not a risk we are prepared to take—and we believe we know how to address that sort of problem. Are 10,000 to perhaps 50,000 wrongfully imprisoned citizens too many? Can we do better? How? There are no obvious answers. The good news is that the great majority of convicted criminal defendants in America are guilty. The bad news is that a substantial number are not.[13]

A Recent Headline: NYPD Boss' Son Returns to TV Show after Rape Claim

> NEW YORK (AP)—The New York City police commissioner's TV host son resumed his morning show duties at "Good Day New York" on Friday, telling viewers it had been a tough couple of weeks but he was ready to get back to work after being cleared of the prospect of criminal charges of raping a woman he met for a drink.
>
> It was Greg Kelly's first day back on the job since he took a leave of absence from the show after the allegations surfaced late last month. . . .
>
> Prosecutors on Tuesday said they had not found cause to charge Kelly with a crime.
>
> The woman told authorities that Kelly raped her in her lower Manhattan office after they went out for drinks on Oct. 8, assaulting her while she wasn't capable of consenting to sex, a person familiar with the investigation said. She told authorities she became pregnant from the encounter and had an abortion, according to a

law enforcement official. Neither the person nor the law official was authorized to speak publicly, and they spoke to The Associated Press on the condition of anonymity.[14]

An earlier AP story provided further details:

> Prosecutors interviewed "numerous relevant fact and expert witnesses," analyzed receipts, security logs, text messages and telephone records and interviewed the woman and Kelly, the chief of the Manhattan district attorney's office sex crimes unit, Martha Bashford, wrote in a letter Tuesday to Kelly's lawyer, Andrew M. Lankler.
>
> "After reviewing all of the evidence, we have determined that the facts established during our investigation do not fit the definitions of sexual assault crimes under New York criminal law," Bashford wrote. "Therefore, no criminal charges are appropriate."
>
> Kelly had vehemently denied doing anything wrong, and he portrayed the prosecutors' conclusions as vindication. . . . The woman, who works at a downtown Manhattan law firm, told police she met Kelly on the street; they then arranged to meet for drinks three days later at a bar at the nearby South Street Seaport, a second person familiar with the investigation has said, speaking on condition of anonymity to discuss details not made public. The woman and Kelly stayed in contact afterward, the first person said.
>
> The woman's boyfriend learned the story and became enraged, that person said.
>
> Before the woman went to police, her boyfriend confronted the commissioner in person at a public event, saying Greg Kelly had ruined his girlfriend's life but declining to elaborate on the spot when asked what he meant, police spokesman Paul Browne said. The commissioner suggested the boyfriend send him a letter, but the man apparently never did, Browne said.
>
> Prosecutors do not plan to charge Kelly's accuser with any crime, DA's office spokeswoman Joan Vollero said.[15]

In May 2012, a Los Angeles Superior Court overturned a forcible rape conviction against Brian Banks after his accuser, Wanetta Gibson, admitted she falsely accused Banks of the crime. Banks was only 17 at the time of his arrest, but was a star high school football player, there was verbal commitment to play college ball at USC and it seemed as if a professional football career was not out of reach. Gibson, who was 15 at the time, claimed she was raped by Banks, he claimed the sex was consensual. Rather than risk a prison term of 41 years to life, he agreed to a plea bargain of five years.

Shortly after this, the Gibson family sued the Long Beach Unified School District for maintaining an unsafe environment. Gibson and her family got 1.5 million dollars.

At the age of 24, Gibson contacted Banks on Facebook and a meeting took place, which was recorded by a private investigator who accompanied Banks. She admitted that the rape charge was false. This became the basis for overturning the conviction in 2012.

The chances of a NFL professional football career as a player seem to be gone, though he has tried out for several teams. An emotional portrayal of the case was aired on the CBS News program *60 Minutes* in March of 2013. Meanwhile, the Los Angeles District Attorney's office has made at the time of this writing, no announcement of any charge of perjury or making a false claim to police officers against Gibson.

An examination of the 1,085 cleared and exonerated cases by the National Registry of Exonerations at the University of Michigan School of Law finds that 223 were charges of sexual assault, or 21 percent of the total. False accusations of child sexual abuse amounted to 132 cases, or 12 percent of the total.[16]

Hang 'Em High?

The American Bar Association in a paper for the ABA Section of Litigation Annual Conference in 2008, referenced the actions of Michael Nifong, the former District Attorney of Durham, North Carolina and the Duke Lacrosse case that led eventually to his disbarment. "Some argue that the situation involving Nifong is an isolated case. Yet, prosecutorial overreaching has been an issue well before this headline-grabbing case came along." The article, "Crossing the Line: Responding to Prosecutorial Misconduct," pointed to a review of more than 2,000 appellate cases in California and verified such misconduct in more than 400:

> Perhaps the most disturbing statistic is that a follow-up study looking at half of the cases resulting in a reversed conviction concluded that the prosecutor was not referred to the California State Bar for discipline, which is required under California law. If there is a positive aspect to the Duke Lacrosse saga, it is that Nifong's actions and ultimate disbarment have served to highlight the important issue of prosecutorial misconduct and

the need for effective remedies . . . Regardless of the causes, the effects of prosecutorial misconduct are distressing. Two different studies of persons exonerated by DNA evidence have shown that prosecutorial misconduct played a role in convicting an innocent person nearly half of the time. . . . Moreover, assuming that the defendant is factually culpable, a conviction secured through the improper actions of a prosecutor could be unconstitutional and, thus, subject to reversal. The result is that the innocent are convicted and the guilty go free, which can only exacerbate the public's loss of trust in the integrity of the criminal justice system.

The ABA report points out that very few prosecutors suffer any consequences: "In January 1999, the *Chicago Tribune* published a five-part series titled: *Trial & Error: How Prosecutors Sacrifice Justice to Win.* Analyzing thousands of cases, the newspaper found that since 1963 at least 381 defendants had their convictions reversed either because prosecutors suppressed exculpatory evidence or suborned perjury." Alarmingly, of those 381 cases, "not one of those prosecutors was convicted of a crime. Not one was barred from practicing law. Instead, many saw their careers advance, becoming judges or district attorneys. One became a congressman."[17]

And, of course, as some judges note, "For someone to falsely accuse another out of anger and vengeance silences the voices of the many real victims."[18] Elaine Epstein, former president of the Massachusetts Bar Association, did speak plainly about what happens at the courthouse—particularly regarding allegations of domestic violence, "Everyone knows that restraining orders and orders to vacate are granted to virtually all who apply. . . . In many cases, allegations of abuse are now used for tactical advantage."[19]

Let us assume, for the moment, that a serious case can be made for the existence of widespread manipulation of the system that results in false allegations, especially regarding the family law system. Let us also assume that the ill effects associated with the phenomena directly impact men more often than women. Let us also assume that many more men are assaulted in general by this type of thing than are ever sexually abused by an adult woman.

What percentage, then, of adult women who sexually abuse men in some form use the tactic of a false allegation to further gain power and control?

We do not know. Certainly, we do not know as a percentage or can give any good estimate of total numbers—not yet. We can, however, begin to answer some initial questions, at least in terms of the anecdotal evidence.

Are false family law allegations more often leveled at men rather than women? Yes, that seems obvious.

Are the false accusations of abuse, either sexual or physical, more readily believed and acted upon by authorities when made by a woman? We do not really know. Would an accusation by a man against a woman for sexually abusing a child be readily listened to by those in authority? I think it would as equally as it would be, coming from a woman against a man. We do know that about a significant percentage of allegations of child sexual abuse are false when made in a divorce/custody battle, but a roughly equal number are true. It is also the "atom bomb" of custody disputes, so not as often used as other false allegation tactics. We can say with some certainty even by looking at police arrest versus survey results that there is a greater likelihood that a woman's complaints of physical assault against an intimate partner are more likely to be believed than the reverse. Many men assume that any allegations of abuse against a woman for any reason, physical or sexual, is less likely to be believed than if a woman was doing it, just because they are a man. This, however, is an assumption that is not entirely proven. It may not be as exceptional an event as is supposed.

In speaking with attorneys, judges, and law enforcement officials about these issues, I find that if presented with sufficient evidence, they will act.

The issue then becomes more focused on information and helping men seek help and assisting their concerned family and friends in doing the same.

Do false allegations also sometimes take the form of sexual abuse?

Absolutely. The sexual harassment that our second letter writer experienced was directly linked to a false allegation. It is quite true that we have no direct measurements for this belief. We only have the anecdotal record, but that is substantial enough to ensure its veracity.

I was especially intrigued by a little gem of a book, *The Morning After-Sex, Fear and Feminism on Campus.*[20] Katie Roiphe, a Princeton University graduate, wrote of her personal experiences on campus and took a look at what was going on at Yale and Harvard as well.

One in Four, One in Five, or None of the Above, and Does It Matter?

Roiphe's examination of events and consequences of the climate at her university and others is worth quoting directly. Not so much for the data that she explores, which has been examined by numerous others and is worth repeating here, but in how she came to examine factually the information that she had been forced-fed on campus: "If I was really standing in the middle of an epidemic, a crisis, if 25 percent of my female friends were really being raped, wouldn't I know it? The answer is not that there is a conspiracy of silence. The answer is that measuring rape is not as straightforward as it seems."

One in four women in college has been the victim of rape or attempted rape. Sometimes, this changed to one in five women. The office of Vice President Joe Biden has released numerous press releases stating that one in five women on campus have been victims of sexual assault. Inflated prevalence of rape claims are also supported by the new CDC survey.

There are several ways of examining the statistic, and readers who want more details should refer to the notes.[21] Perhaps the best way to put it into perspective is to do the math, rather than delve into the awful details of how badly the highly questionable "research" was skewed to reach a desired result and inflated numbers. It is edifying to note that to get to one in four rapes on college campus, 73 percent of the women whom the researcher (Koss) characterized as rape victims said that they had not been raped. Forty-three percent of the supposed victims had intercourse again with their alleged assailants, yet they were "raped." This was all from a 1987 survey by Koss that received widespread attention and the subsequent intuition of services to deal with the "epidemic" and "crisis."

In the latest variation, the one in five women on campus will be a victim of sexual assault also includes such assaults as consisting of "a forced kiss." Despite the labels when the results of this survey are looked at in detail, we find that only 3 percent of the women questioned said they experienced physical or psychological harm. Only 2 percent reported what happened to authorities. Thirty-six percent said it was not clear any crime or harm had been committed, and 66 percent said they did not report the incident because it was not serious enough. Fully half of the respondents who advocates claim had been sexually assaulted said that they were partially or fully responsible for what happened.

The real versus the unreal, however, gives us a better picture than criticism over research methods, conclusions, and their interpretation by advocates—writing in *City Journal*, journalist Heather Mac Donald notes that, "The 2006 violent crime rate in Detroit, one of the most violent cities in America, was 2,400 murders, rapes, robberies, and aggravated assaults per 100,000 inhabitants—a rate of 2.4 percent. The one-in-four statistic would mean that every year, millions of young women graduate who have suffered the most terrifying assault, short of murder, that a woman can experience."[22] "If the one-in-four statistic is correct—it is sometimes modified to one-in-five—campus rape represents a crime wave of unprecedented proportions. No crime, much less one as serious as rape, has a victimization rate remotely approaching 20 or 25 percent, even over many years."[23] *Philadelphia Magazine* writer Sandy Hingston, also did some math: "Take Temple University. There are 30,000 students at its main campus. The student body is 55 percent female, so if the one-in-five Department of Justice figure for sexual assaults is correct, 3,180 of the current female students would have been sexually assaulted while at the school. And yet Temple's Cleary Act report shows five sexual assaults in 2007, two in 2008, and two in 2009."[24]

The 1987 one-in-four claim first published in *Ms. Magazine*, Mac Donald points out, "took the universities by storm." She gives a succinct picture of what happened next:

> By the early 1990s, campus rape centers and 24-hour hotlines were opening across the country, aided by tens of millions of dollars of federal funding. Victimhood rituals sprang up: first the Take Back the Night rallies, in which alleged rape victims reveal their stories to gathered crowds of candle-holding supporters; then the Clothes-line Project, in which T-shirts made by self-proclaimed rape survivors are strung on campus, while recorded sounds of gongs and drums mark minute-by-minute casualties of the "rape culture." A special rhetoric emerged: victims' family and friends were "co-survivors"; "survivors" existed in a larger "community of survivors."
>
> An army of salesmen took to the road, selling advice to administrators on how to structure sexual-assault procedures, and lecturing freshmen on the "undetected rapists" in their midst. Rape bureaucrats exchanged notes at such gatherings as the Inter Ivy Sexual Assault Conferences and the New England College Sexual Assault Network. Organizations like One in Four and Men Can Stop Rape tried to persuade college boys to redefine their masculinity away from the "rape culture." The college rape infrastructure shows no signs of a slowdown. In 2006, for example, Yale created a new Sexual Harassment and Assault Resources and Education Center, despite numerous resources for rape victims already on campus.[25]

A Climate of Fear = A Hostile Work Environment

Our effort here is to examine ways in which adult men are sometimes sexually abused by adult women, and in some sense by adult men who support abusive women, at least in political or social terms. It is not to engage in a general debate over statistics and how they are used or misused. How misinformation and the unreasoning fear it can create works is what we want to examine, and more importantly, how that can affect individuals in an adverse way is what we seek to explore.

One might debate and even discount the effect of campus policies and "take back the night" rallies and even doubt that they have much impact on most students, even male ones. But, it is getting a lot more serious—fast.

The New Department of Education Directive

U.S. Department of Education rules now force persons to abandon their due process rights in order to get an education. They are considered guilty until proven innocent whenever an on-campus sexual accusation occurs. On April 4, 2011, the DED Office of Civil Rights (OCR) instructed every university that accepts federal funds to use a "preponderance (51%) of evidence" standard in evaluating allegations of sexual offense, including rape. An accuser only needs to "tip the scales" for a professor or student to be found "guilty."

The American Association of University Professors (AAUP) did object. The group wants sexual accusations to be judged by a higher standard than traffic courts use for parking tickets.

On June 27, Gregory Scholtz, AAUP's Director of the Department of Academic Freedom, Tenure, and Governance wrote to DED to protest the "lower standard of proof" that threatens "academic freedom and tenure."

Then, on August 18, 2011, AAUP's Chair of the Committee on Women expressed concern about the "potential for accusations, even false ones, to ruin a faculty member's career." Backlash from two separate units of the AAUP is remarkable. Their recognition of false accusations is extraordinary.

As a result of the DED directive, campuses are already beginning to reverse the presumption of innocence. Based on questionable data, men are assumed to be predators and women are said to "never lie" about issues such as rape. By lowering the standards of justice, the OCR is encouraging false accusations.

The Department of Education's "Dear Colleague" directive issued on April 4, 2011 leaves no room for a school to deviate from the "preponderance of the evidence" standard. It states in clear and unequivocal terms "Thus, in order for a school's grievance procedures to be consistent with Title IX standards, the school must use a pre-ponderance of the evidence standard (i.e., *it is more likely than not* [emphasis added] that sexual harassment or violence occurred)." If the school does not follow the DED rule, the penalty can be severe—loss of federal funds.

People lie for many reasons, including revenge and shame; people also make mistakes. This is why courts presume an accused to be innocent and place the burden of proof on the accuser. Hard evidence and due process are all the more important in sexual cases that often devolve to "he said, she said."

On campus at least, a climate of fear has definitely been created. It is not just an isolated case such as that of the Duke Lacrosse players, which works its way into the national headlines. One must recall that over 60 faculty members rushed to judgment in that case in a full page campus newspaper ad. To date, none have publically apologized or taken out an ad to do so, when the players were later vindicated. It does not seem to matter that their lives and those of every other member of their team were deeply adversely affected.

Mac Donald gives us several more cases with real-life effects on men:

In October 2005, at a Delta Delta formal, drunken sorority girls careened through the host's house, vomiting, falling, and breaking furnishings. One girl ran naked through a hallway; another was found half-naked with a male on the bed in the master suite. A third had intercourse with her escort in a different bedroom. On the bus back from the formal, she was seen kissing her escort; once she arrived home, she had sex with a different male. Later, she accused her escort of rape. The district attorney declined to prosecute the girl's rape charges. William and Mary, however, had already forced the defendant to leave school and, even after the D.A.'s decision, wouldn't let him return until his accuser graduated. The defendant sued his accuser for $5.5 million for defamation; the parties settled out of court.

The incident wasn't as unusual as it sounds. A year earlier, a William and Mary student had charged rape after having provided a condom to her partner for intercourse. The boy had cofounded the national anti-rape organization One in Four; the school suspended him for a year, anyway. In an earlier incident, a drunken sorority girl was filmed giving oral sex to seven men. She cried rape when her boyfriend found out. William and Mary found one of the recipients, who had taped the event, guilty of assault and suspended him.[26]

If the Department of Education rule stands up to legal challenge, we can expect many more such incidents on campus; this October 2011 case is but one example, as reported by the organization, FIRE:

> A student convicted of sexual assault and banned from campus by a University of North Dakota (UND) tribunal is free to return to school. After a year and a half, UND officials have determined that the university's finding of guilt against student Caleb Warner was "not substantiated" in the face of the evidence. That same evidence led North Dakota law enforcement to charge Warner's accuser last year with making a false report to law enforcement—a charge for which she is still wanted by the police. UND finally reexamined Warner's case only after the university's behavior was exposed by the Foundation for Individual Rights in Education (FIRE), to which Warner had turned for help.
>
> "Using a shamefully low standard of evidence, the University of North Dakota branded Caleb Warner a criminal. Meanwhile, based on the very same evidence, law enforcement officials charged Warner's accuser with lying to them and issued a warrant for her arrest," said FIRE President Greg Lukianoff. "Cases like this vividly demonstrate the need for due process and fair procedure on campus, as well as a renewed recognition that fundamental rights are important for both victims and the accused."
>
> In finding Warner guilty, UND used the weak "preponderance of the evidence" standard (50.01% certainty) to determine guilt or innocence—the very same standard recently imposed upon every federally funded college in the country under an April 2011 regulation from the federal Department of Education's Office for Civil Rights.[27]

It is also clear that even if the regulation does not remain in effect, the backing of the vice president of the United States and other strong entities who will remain, regardless of political fortunes, assures a robust future for campus kangaroo courts, as will the CDC survey of one in five women "raped." "Universities are equipped to handle plagiarism, not rape," observes University of Pennsylvania history professor Alan Charles Kors. "Sexual-assault charges, if true, are so serious as to belong only in the criminal system."[28]

Mac Donald adds, "New York University's Wellness Exchange counsels people to 'believe unconditionally' in sexual-assault charges because 'only 2 percent of reported rapes are false reports'" (a ubiquitous claim that dates from radical feminist Susan Brownmiller's 1975 tract *Against Our Will*). As Stuart Taylor and K.C. Johnson point out in their book *Until Proven Innocent*, however, the rate of false reports is at least 9 percent and probably closer to 50 percent. Just how powerful is the "believe unconditionally" credo? David Lisak, a University of Massachusetts psychology professor who lectures constantly on the anti-rape college circuit, acknowledged to a hall of Rutgers students that the "Duke case," in which a stripper falsely accused three Duke lacrosse players of rape in 2006, "has raised the issue of false allegations." But Lisak did not want to talk about the Duke case, he said. "I don't know what happened at Duke. No one knows." Actually, we do know what happened at Duke—the prosecutor ignored clearly exculpatory evidence and alibis that cleared the defendants, and was later disbarred for his misconduct. But to the campus rape industry, a lying plaintiff remains a victim of the patriarchy, and the accused remain forever under suspicion. It also of course, places young women in the position of never being responsible for their own actions, as Mac Donald points out:

> The baby boomers who demanded the dismantling of all campus rules governing the relations between the sexes now sit in dean's offices and student-counseling services. They cannot turn around and argue for reregulating sex, even on pragmatic grounds. Instead, they have responded to the fallout of the college sexual revolution with bizarre and anachronistic legalism. Campuses have created a judicial infrastructure for responding to post coital second thoughts more complex than that required to adjudicate maritime commerce claims in Renaissance Venice.
>
> Even if the . . . victim's drunkenness cancels any responsibility that she might share for the interaction's finale, is she equally without responsibility for all of her behavior up to that point, including getting so drunk that she can't remember anything? Campus rape ideology holds that inebriation strips women of responsibility for their actions but preserves male responsibility not only for their own actions but for their partners' as well. . . .
>
> Modern feminists defined the right to be promiscuous as a cornerstone of female equality. Understandably, they now hesitate

to acknowledge that sex is a more complicated force than was foreseen. Rather than recognizing that no-consequences sex may be a contradiction in terms, however, the campus rape industry claims that what it calls campus rape is not about sex but rather politics—the male desire to subordinate women. The University of Virginia Women's Center intones that "rape or sexual assault is not an act of sex or lust—it's about aggression, power, and humiliation, using sex as the weapon. The rapist's goal is domination."

This characterization may or may not describe the psychopathic violence of stranger rape. But it is an absurd description of the barnyard rutting that undergraduate men, happily released from older constraints, seek. The guys who push themselves on women at keggers are after one thing only, and it's not a reinstatement of the patriarchy. Each would be perfectly content if his partner for the evening becomes president of the United States one day, so long as she lets him take off her panties tonight.[29]

In the *Philadelphia Magazine* article, Hingston agrees:

Administrators warn that even with the guidelines, campus hearing boards are ill-equipped to investigate assaults and rapes—all in the midst of *another* epidemic, binge drinking. Peter F. Lake, director of the Center for Excellence in Higher Education Law and Policy at Stetson University, told the *Chronicle of Higher Education*, "We've been lured into doing something in a criminal justice model that the criminal justice system itself hasn't been able to deal with. . . ."

At precisely the time in their lives when young men and women should be exploring what sexuality means, the new rules choke off their freedom, limit their choices, and encourage the canard that all males are unrepentant predators. What's more, they position women as helpless victims who require bureaucratic protection from those males—victims with no responsibility for their own behavior. Heaven help those women when they graduate.[30]

In an opinion article published in the *Wall Street Journal,* Peter Berkowitz, PhD, JD and a senior fellow at the Hoover Institution, titled his article, "Sex Smears and the Rule of Law at Yale."

The case of former Yale quarterback Patrick Witt provides additional evidence, as if more were needed, that our leading colleges and universities have lost their way.

Controversy erupted on Jan. 26, when the *New York Times* tarnished the reputation of Yale's star football player. According to reporter Richard Pérez-Peña, Mr. Witt, a finalist for a prestigious Rhodes Scholarship, did not withdraw from the scholarship competition in November because, as he claimed at the time, he preferred to lead his team against Harvard in "The Game" instead of flying to Atlanta for his scheduled Rhodes interview.

Rather, according to Mr. Pérez-Peña, the Rhodes committee, having "learned through unofficial channels that a fellow student had accused Witt of sexual assault," suspended his candidacy until such time as Yale provided a letter re-endorsing it.

Mr. Witt has denied the charge, and the Times story has been harshly criticized. The Times reported the existence of a confidential accusation of sexual assault despite not knowing the name of the accuser or the content of the complaint. . . .

The complaint lodged against Mr. Witt was part of a new system for dealing with sexual-assault accusations at Yale . . . (Mr. Berkowitz goes on to explain in detail the new Department of Education directive which Yale like other colleges are bound to follow or lose federal funds) . . . The Patrick Witt case, which is not atypical, reflects more than the decline of due process on campus. It also exhibits a failure of liberal education . . . If Yale and other institutions across the country were fulfilling their promise to educate students, then their faculties would teach that riding roughshod over due process shows ignorance of or contempt for the rule of law . . . The need to restore due process on campus-and in the directives of the federal government-is urgent.[31]

Broader Implications

Readers may question the emphasis here on the campus picture to the exclusion of effects on men to similar efforts in other parts of society. As we have stated, however, the research is severely limited beyond this population, and even so, it is scanty within it, certainly in comparison to the research regarding sexual assaults, harassment, and stalking against females. This book, we hope, will raise questions, and just as importantly, encourage more research.

The results of what happens on campuses do affect everyone ultimately. In a 2003 essay published in the book *Abuse Your Illusions*[32] titled, "The Mysterious Decline of Men on Campus," this author (Cook) and columnist Glenn Sacks were among the first to point to a trend that shows no signs of declining; in fact, it is growing. Females now outnumber males by a four-to-three ratio, a difference of almost two million students. In 2009, for every 100 men, 142 women graduated with a bachelors, 159 women completed masters and 107 women got a doctoral degree.[33] According to the U.S. Department of Education, in 1971, the percentages of men outnumbered women in degrees conferred 61 to 39, but by 2017, expect a complete reversal.

Women's studies textbooks provide a view of the hostility towards men in our universities. According to an extensive study of women's studies textbooks released in 2002 by the Independent Women's Foundation, a dissident women's group, the textbooks "ignore facts in favor of myths," "mistake ideology for scholarship," and encourage students to "embrace aggrievement, not knowledge."[34] The study, "Lying in a Room of One's Own: How Women's Studies Textbooks Miseducate Students," examined the five most popular Women Studies' textbooks in the United States and found relentless woman-as-victim/man-as-victimizer bias and hostility. According to the author, Christine Stolba, the textbooks construe or distort studies and statistics to infer that women are miserable and oppressed, and that men are privileged oppressors.[35]

Among the "truths" the textbooks tell students are—women are under siege from virtually all sectors of society; little has changed for women in the past three decades; believing that women have achieved equality is "modern sexism"; and most women are not naturally sexually attracted to men but are the victims of "compulsory heterosexuality" maintained through male "social control."[36] Bad fathers are described as the rule rather than the exception, the prevalence of sexual abuse and molestation is wildly exaggerated, and students are told that in families, fathers often represent a "foreign male element" that mothers and daughters must unite against.[37]

UCLA is one of the few universities in which a debate on the anti-male bias on campus has actually been allowed to take place, and this was only because of a full-page ad in the campus newspaper. The Independent Women's Forum (IWF) ran a full-page advertisement in UCLA's student newspaper, the *Daily Bruin*, which asked "Are you tired of male-bashing and victimology?" The ad debunked what it called the "Ten Most Common Feminist Myths," including "30 percent of emergency room visits by women each year are the result of injuries from domestic violence," "women have been shortchanged in medical research," "one in four women in college has been the victim of rape or attempted rape," and others.[38] Feminists, led by Tina Oakland, director of the UCLA Center for Women and Men, and Christie Scott, executive co-chair of the UCLA Clothesline Project, launched campus demonstrations against what Scott called "a violent ad, a very hostile ad" that "breeds a very bad attitude toward campus women."[39] Oakland said that challenging one in four is like denying the Holocaust. A feminist professor wrote to the *Daily Bruin* claiming that the IWF ad served to "ferment intolerant, anti-woman . . . sentiment and action on campus" and "incite hate."[40] While the *Daily Bruin* refused to apologize for the ad, its viewpoint editor was cowed, and expressed regret that the paper had "let something so anti-woman through."[41] Oakland, after being castigated by some in conservative magazines, backed off of her defense of the "1 in 4" figure rape figure, explaining that "the statistics don't really matter that much in the big picture."[42]

Can Balance Be Achieved?

A serious national effort is needed to redress the gender imbalance in our universities and the biggest solution to the absence of boys from our college campuses will be boy-friendly reforms at the K-12 level. Christina Hoff Sommers notes that one of the greatest challenges reformers face is the fact that our society is largely unaware of or refuses to recognize the boy crisis in our schools. She contrasts this with England, which embarked upon boy-friendly educational reforms in the early 90s and has met with some success.[43]

Part of this national effort will be a retooling of our schools to create boy-friendly classrooms and teaching strategies. Boys, in particular, need strong, charismatic teachers who mix firm discipline with a good-natured acceptance of boyish energy. Concomitantly, a sharp increase in the number of male teachers is also needed, particularly at the elementary level, where female teachers outnumber male teachers six to one. Same-sex classes may also be helpful, and schools should have the power to employ them when appropriate.[44]

Beyond reforms at the K–12 level, it is apparent that college campuses need to be places where males feel as welcome as females. Women's Studies as a particular course of study should, in fact, be abolished. The proper place to study gender and sex is in established more rigorous academic disciplines, for example, sociology, history, psychology, biology, anthropology, medicine, and the law. I will make the offer here to publically debate the issue: "Resolved the Women's Studies Department at _____ should be abolished" at any college with such a department. If the experience of other authors of my acquaintance is any guide, however, such an offer is not likely to be accepted. At the least, such departments should be converted to Gender Studies as their title (in reality, not just a name) and its texts and studies put under strict peer review, or departments of equal stature and funding need to be created that are devoted to Men's Studies. It only seems fair and balanced. At the very least, many Women's Studies textbooks need to be replaced by texts that consider both male and female points of view on gender issues and which cite only academically credible research.

If one doubts that there is fierce opposition to any kind of support for men on campus, this article by Toronto-based writer Robyn Urback in the *National Post* detailing a 2012 "controversy" at Simon Fraser University in British Columbia provides perspective. The student union voted to fund a men's center on campus. Urback in her article, points out that as in the United States, such centers are a rarity. In fact, she could find only one other in Canada at the University of Manitoba. Nearly every college campus in both countries has a woman's center. The one at Simon Fraser University was established in 1974 with a budget of $30,000 and the student union decided to fund the new men's center for the same amount. Urback detailed the reaction from the established women's center (centre), noting that they opposed it on the grounds that "The men's centre is everywhere else," and that such a program would only be acceptable if it challenged "popular conceptions about masculinity, confronting homophobia, sexism, racism, classism, and ability issues." They feared that such a masculine space would be actively used in a terrible manner: "We are not interested in seeing a group or centre develop that promotes the status quo, encourages sexual assault, or fosters an atmosphere of competition and violence." The women's center website also declared that: "We know that many men are concerned with the way masculinity denigrates women by making them into sexual objects, is homophobic, encourages violence, and discourages emotional expression."[45] The Women's Centre website linked the opening of such a program to the idea that it would promote violence more than eight times.

Urback offered her views in this manner, saying the opposition to the idea of a men's space on campus proves the need for it:

> Several other students have taken a more direct approach, compiling their objections to the Men's Centre in widely-circulated five-minute YouTube video. One woman with seemingly impeccable foresight declares that, "The Men's Centre will end up being a place to celebrate hegemonic masculinity." She later attacks the credibility of the Centre's proponents, scoffing that they have, "no

experience being in a gender-studies class." . . . Another cautions that the project risks creating a "heteronormative space," while yet another critical male dismisses the Men's Centre as simply, "a room with a PS3 and a bunch of douchebags playing games."

Bravo, students. In your attempt to decry the proposed Men's Centre on all of its supposed merits, you have effectively demonstrated why such a space is so very necessary . . . Judging by the crass sociology catch phrases in the aforementioned video, the consensus is that young men don't need community resources or support. That is a myth.

While statistics show that comparatively, far fewer university-aged men are diagnosed with depression than women, the rate of suicide among men is four times as great. It's not hard to connect the dots: men are suffering in silence. . . .

Men, like women, struggle with issues of victimization, anxiety, and depression, but they must battle in addition with a societal expectation of stoicism. In short—it's not manly to talk about your feelings. And it's precisely for that reason that a Men's Centre on campus is such a necessary initiative.

If brought to fruition, the Men's Centre at SFU might also come with additional boons; namely, the latent effect of debunking some of the prejudicial, discriminatory, and misandrous views (see kids? I can play too) so blatantly expressed in the YouTube video.[46]

The decline in male attendance and college achievement does not appear to be a statistical aberration, or one that will correct itself without attention being paid to the issue. Certainly, society is not better off if a significant number of our best and brightest young men fail to seek or earn a college education. We need to take the first step by acknowledging that the decline of males on campus is a significant social and economic problem. This realization need not detract from the mission to provide equal educational opportunities for women. It may lead to recognizing that at least some real discriminatory lack of accommodation for males in education exists, and that reforms and different approaches are needed. If these steps are not taken, it seems clear that the decline of males on campus will continue at its present rapid rate.[47]

If indeed the college environment today represents a hostile work environment for males, and we conclude it does in many respects, and this environmental ethic permeates itself into the policies, structures, and belief system of authorities dealing with the broader public, as it so often has, then we have a problem that does indeed adversely affect us all.

Sexual Harassment—Proposed Solutions

Warren Farrell argues against any kind of sexual harassment legislation, saying "When today's feminists are proponents of protective legislation, they oppose equality. Sexual Harassment legislation is sexist because it makes only the male responsible for the male role in the sexual dance. It protects the woman who is sexual without protecting coworkers from a woman who would use her sexuality for unearned advancement; nor does it protect the company from this woman. Ultimately, it ignores women's role and therefore ignores women. Except as victim."[48]

Farrell, however, it must be noted, is writing this in 1993. I get the sense that he hoped his message would resonate and cause a reevaluation of the approach.

He urges communication strategy teaching and instruction that is sensitive to the differing styles of women and men, rather than lawsuits, regulations, and legislation.

For many years, Nordstrom stores had a 3 × 5 inch employee manual postcard with one rule: "Nordstrom Rules: Rule #1: Use best judgment in all situations. There will be no additional rules."

Of course, the employee manual today for Nordstrom now runs to about 10 pages and covers a number of issues, including its specific sexual harassment policy.[49]

It is going to be very difficult to turn back the clock, but history does give us a guide. In the 2011, Ken Burns PBS documentary *Prohibition*, the most frequent observation of historians and other commenters on that national mistake was that you cannot legislate morality.

We have documented that there is a definite increase in the number of men filing sexual harassment claims against women. This may well represent a growing feeling and acted upon ethic that "what's good for the goose is good for the gander." We expect this ethic to increase in the future and reveal itself in a number of ways, not the least of which is a reevaluation of work place behavior and attitudes.

That future can be rocky or benign. We are familiar with a recent memo from the executive of a large government agency that sought to bring employee attention to the agencies dress code and its relationship to sexual harassment policy. It started in a casual fashion with "We're all adults here and should act like it." The memo went on to re-state the policy that was felt to be necessary because of some recent complaints (implied in the memo, but not stated as being from women about how other women were dressing, especially on "casual Fridays").

Are we all becoming more sensitive to sexual transgressions in the work place? There is little doubt. The days of the boss chasing the secretary around the desk and other manifestations of sexual harassment have not ended, but surely there has been considerable and verifiable amelioration of such behavior, which indicates that men as well have served notice that some types of sexual aggression toward them in the workplace will also not be tolerated. Have we reached equilibrium where men and women can work freely together and yet still have the opportunity as they had in the past to find a potential mate? Probably not. Certainly, that opportunity is considerably diluted and there is great acceptance of that fact from both women and men. Will the majority of men still have to pursue and women decide? Will such pursuits and reactions still frequently happen in the work place? Most likely. Have such pursuits and decisions taken on a much more cautious atmosphere in the work place? Without a doubt.

We do not purport here to engage in the most dangerous of activities—predicting the future. It does however, seem that our society is moving toward rather than away from a rather balanced approach. Like it or not, old high school rules apply to adults in the work place today. Women may not have to kneel on the gym floor to see if their skirts are long enough to touch the floor, but the effect of dress codes for example, is mainly aimed at them. Other types of sexual harassment rules seem to be more equally gender applicable.

The commentators in *Prohibition* are not wrong in saying that it is impossible to effectively enact legislation to control morality, but if a majority of citizens support such legislation *and* eventually see tangible benefits from it, then moral behavior can be legislated or regulated. The sexual harassment laws and subsequent corporate policies in this regard are such an example.

The tricky part is finding that balance between legislative laws, court interpretation of the law, corporate policy, and common sense. The application of adult sexual harassment laws and policies to the very young in schools is a particularly troubling development. However, we can be assured that sexually harassing behavior in the workplace, despite excesses in the application of rules, and the increased potential for false allegations as an instrument of power and control, is less likely to occur. It is less likely to occur to women, but it also less likely to occur to men.

In the Supreme Court case, *Meritor Savings Bank v. Vinson* in 1986, the court determined that for sexual harassment to be actionable, it must be sufficiently severe or pervasive to alter the conditions of employment and create an abusive working environment.

Corporations and their advisors, however, despite what the ruling said, have moved to take action even when the complaint does not rise to the severe or pervasive levels or the creation of an abusive environment.

In an article called, "A New Era in Sexual Harassment," Mauricio Velasquez, of the Diversity Training Group, says that corporations must be aware that it happens to men as well, but steps can be taken to provide protection both for corporations and individual employees:

> The most prominent of the new age complaints are those cases involving men harassed by female supervisors . . . Men represent 10% of all sexual harassment cases and the numbers are steadily rising. In most harassment cases, whether the assailant is male or female, the main motive is not romance but power. Today, women hold 15% of all managerial and supervisory positions and are now more than ever inclined to play the power game. However, females tend to differ from males in their demands. When a male becomes a victim of sexual harassment by a female, more than 50% of the cases allege a demand for sex—Quid Pro Quo—in order to retain a job or receive a promotion. By contrast, quid pro quo is only evident in 15% of female victim's cases. The main dilemma a man faces when he is harassed by a woman is that he is more inclined to be embarrassed and is reluctant to speak out for fear that he will be humiliated and ostracized by his coworkers. Male victim cases can sometimes present problems due to society's stereotypes of women and men. Our mental models maintain the assumption that males find sexual advances from women non-threatening and even enjoyable.
>
> We must take all complaints seriously or we will lose creditability. Procedures for dealing with harassment cases should be consistent, regardless of gender or status. However, companies should still take into account the victim's personality and the circumstances. They should treat every complaint confidentially, investigate each thoroughly and take appropriate and immediate disciplinary action.[50]

James Taranto writes a column for the *Wall Street Journal*, mainly the online version at WSJ.com. The accusations against presidential candidate Herman Cain were in the news, and as many commentators and news organizations did during this period, Taranto took the opportunity to comment and he began it with an email from a reader:

> In the first incident, we were in a team meeting. One female member came late. The seats were all taken. Our CEO says to her that as there are no chairs, she is welcome to sit in his lap . . . Later in the same meeting, he compliments her on her dress and says something to the effect that the dress probably looks even better off of her . . . She goes to file an action against him and the chief operating officer says basically: Everyone knows he's a jackass. Get over it. Rather than get over it, she gets an attorney. There is a brief investigation, our board has a Saturday morning phone conference, and by Saturday afternoon we are looking for a new CEO and a new COO.
>
> In the second incident, I had hired a new manager. One of his staff had wanted the job . . . She welcomed him by refusing to do every assignment he gave her. He and I met with the head of human resources and developed her "performance improvement plan." . . . She left the meeting, went to HR and said he called her a whore and fondled himself during the session. . . . The investigation— bringing in every female in the office and asking if he had ever made them uncomfortable or said anything untoward—ripped him apart. He was cleared, and the accuser left before she got fired. But he never got over it.[51]

Taranto offered these on-point comments following his printing of the email from the reader:

> These two stories neatly illustrate both the necessity for sexual harassment laws and the injustice of the way they are currently applied . . . Two comments in one meeting might have fallen short of the quantitative standard of pervasiveness. Still, it was undoubtedly wise of the board to fire the pair. In this case, the system worked. . . .
>
> In the second case, however, the accused man was innocent. The system also "worked" in that he was not fired or formally punished. But the investigation itself was agonizing . . . In a just world she would have been summarily fired for making an accusation that executives knew to be false.

The fallen nature of man is gender-neutral. Some men are pigs, and some women are liars. Current sexual harassment law deals justly and effectively with the former at the cost of allowing the latter to do great harm to innocent men. The presence of both sexes in the workplace makes necessary some combination of laws, policies and customs to regulate sexual behavior on the job. But the principle of heads-she-wins-tails-he-loses does violence to both justice and equality.[52]

We believe that the opportunity for proper training with gender-sensitive and gender-inclusive components that is available to corporations, businesses, and government agencies that can afford it is certainly a key part of the solution towards common sense. We cannot, unfortunately, get by anymore with just the postcard-sized Nordstrom employee manual as much as we might wish to, but we can do a much better job of making sure that frivolous, mean-spirited and self-serving false accusations are met with the same condemnation and even the same legal and professional consequences as the actual practice of sexual harassment.

Stalking—Proposed Approaches

The dictum in our chapter on stalking that victims must "document, document, document," remains the best advice. Smartphones and other video and audio recording devices, as well as keeping copies of emails and other forms of communication, are the first line of defense. If you can prove the case to officials with such records, it is a lot easier to get action. After such documentation is made, then police can take a report, be on the lookout for the stalker, give warnings to the stalker, and even make arrests.

Restraining/protective orders form the next line of defense. They are easy to get and do not require an attorney. They are perhaps too easy to get, and judges should be cautious when such orders involve live-in intimate partners or spouses, especially when custody issues and substantial property is involved. Stranger or former intimate stalking restraining/protective orders should be a fairly straightforward legal remedy. Victims, however, should not expect that the mere existence of such an order will solve all problems. Indeed, for truly violent or disturbed individuals, such orders may increase the danger to the victim. They do not lead to an immediate arrest, but only arrest a person found to be in violation of the order and need to be renewed every year.

In particular, it seems for males, as we have shown in the chapter, they must be more cautious than they show a propensity for, in revealing personal details on the internet. Internet security experts say such precautions must form the first line of defense. All the technical security in the world, though necessary, will not prevent cyber stalking if personal details are posted on the internet or sensitive information such as passwords are revealed by the target. That is how a case of cyber stalking usually starts. The Washington case reported by the television station of the women's magazine editor was a "successful" alleged stalking because the perpetrator had a given out or allowed her to obtain, his password, which then gave her access to his personal and business email addresses.

Stalking can also be an area where false allegations are not as rare as one might suspect. In *Criminal Justice and Behavior*, a study found the rate of false reporting to be nearly 12 percent, out of 357 reported claims.[53] In *Ethical Human Psychology and Psychiatry*, investigators of such false stalking claims found that the majority of such reporters were delusional (64%), while the remainder were evenly divided between the attention seeker, and hypersensitivity to previous victimization by stalking, with a small category (7%) being the stalker themselves.[54]

Thus, caution should be a by-word for those in authority investigating stalking claims, while at the same time, such claims made by men, must be taken as seriously as they would be if made by a woman against a man.

Rape and Sexual Assault

Language

The largest anti-rape organization is RAINN-Rape Abuse Incest National Network.[55] They have a toll-free hotline, other resources, and a prominent website. They appear to be gender-inclusive in most of their statements: "Anyone may be a victim of rape: women, *men* or children, straight or gay." However, there are several instances in their literature, where they miss the boat. For example, in the way they frame a commonly asked question on their website, "And I was drunk, or *he* was drunk—does that mean it isn't rape?" There is nothing wrong with the response, but the question asked applies only to women and not a man. RAINN could have framed the same question in a gender-inclusive way, but they failed to do so. The organization needs to review all of their information and make certain that *every* statement is gender-inclusive.

While it is impossible to review every rape crisis victim advocacy or helpline site in the world to review their statements for gender-inclusive language, the cursory review we have conducted indicates that the RAINN site is likely to be not typical, but actually better than most.

We appreciate the New York University (NYU) website about the same issues and giving out much of the same advice, but it is a website that uses gender-inclusive language throughout: "A hospital will store the rape kit for 30 days, which allows for the survivor to later decide if *she/he* wants to report to the police . . . If the survivor does not choose to have a rape kit completed, *she/he* also has the option to . . ."[56]

The NYU website further points out that, "States must certify that they do not require a victim of sexual assault to participate in the criminal justice system or cooperate with law enforcement in order to be provided with a forensic medical exam, reimbursement for charges incurred on account of such an exam, or both. Under this law, a state must ensure that victims have access to an exam free of charge or with a full reimbursement, even if the victim decides not to cooperate with law enforcement."

This is very useful information for victims, whether they are male or female.

Information about Erections and Ejaculation

The NYU website in a clear and direct manner, addresses some common concerns of male victims:

> Can rape happen to "real men?"
> Rape is something that can and does happen to an entire spectrum of men, regardless of physical strength or prowess. Being raped does not mean that the survivor is weak or a wimp. Anyone can be overpowered or taken by surprise. Size and strength is often no match for weapons, overwhelming odds, or a surprise attack.
> Can a man still have an erection if he is frightened?
> All studies so far have found that survivors commonly do report erections and even ejaculations while being raped. These are uncontrollable, automatic, physiological responses, and do not mean that the survivor enjoyed the experience.[57]

It must also be remembered that some women report that lubrication occurred even though they were being violently raped.

This is the most common question put first to the authors by a few initial media interviews. There will be many more such interviews to come once this volume is published. It is without a doubt, the most common question. The best response perhaps is with another question:

"If I stepped hard on your toe right now—what would you say?" The answer from the interviewer is always, "Well, I would say, 'ouch.'" They are then asked if they could have prevented themselves from saying "ouch?" The interviewer then admits that they probably could not have prevented themselves from saying "ouch" even when they knew in advance that their toe was about to be stepped on. We then point out that saying "ouch" is an automatic physical response and control is either not possible or very limited. We go on to explain that it is the same with men, given stimulation, a significant number of male rape victims will experience an erection, similarly, a significant percentage of female rape victims report lubrication. It does not mean the experience was enjoyable, that they were not in fear, in distress or did not want to have sex, or that they were not raped. We also point out that in the cases of males, objects are often used by women for anal rape. Even oral sex when the man objects, or is too incapacitated to object, is rape of a sort, or at the least, sexual assault.

It should also be pointed out that some rapists *intend* to cause ejaculation, which can be an involuntary response to stimuli. The intention of the rapist is to demonstrate power and control—*See, I made you do this*—as well as act as bulwark against any accusation that may result from her actions. *He came—so he must have enjoyed it—therefore, it wasn't rape or sexual assault.*

Surviving as a Male

This author conducted a lengthy interview with Howard Fradkin, PhD, LICDC a co-founder of malesurvivor.org. He has counseled over 1,000 male survivors in individual, couples, group psychotherapy, and weekend workshops over the course of his 28-year career as a psychologist. As co-chairperson of the MaleSurvivor Weekends of Recovery, Fradkin has directed 34 Weekends of Recovery since 2001 for over 600 men. Dr. Fradkin has also supervised and trained hundreds of professional colleagues on the topic of psychotherapy with male survivors of sexual abuse. 1in6.org is another prominent organization in this arena, but it is focused almost exclusively on childhood trauma, and thus not the best resource for males who experience sexual abuse as an adult from another adult. Fradkin is particularly proud that the organization's conferences are open not only to professionals, but also to survivors. The website is accessed by about a million unique visitors a year.

Awareness and the Media

He notes that considerable progress has been made in terms of basic information. Particularly, he says, in the most critical piece—the acknowledgement that males can indeed be victims of sexual abuse. Certainly, he sees progress in terms of a greater awareness that males can be victims of childhood sexual abuse, though of course, more needs to be done.

He calls the idea that adult women can sexually abuse men as, "One of the most shameful and privately kept secrets out there for men. The idea that men can be abused by a woman is very difficult for any man who has been victimized to acknowledge and get help for. So, the fact that you are writing this book is huge. It is the biggest piece of information that is not out there, that women are capable of abusing men. That it has nothing to do with how strong a man is, how masculine he is, how virile he is-men can be victimized."[58]

Fradkin says that he sees a lot of progress in the past few years in terms of media acknowledgment, and points to an Oprah Winfrey show as indicative when the story of Tyler Perry's childhood victimization—by men and women—was detailed and the general subject was discussed. But even there, he "had to argue with the producers who initially only wanted to do a show about men who were victimized only by men." But he was successful in convincing the producers that this would be a huge disservice. He says it takes courage by the news media to tell the truth about female perpetrators and male victims because they are "fearful of being labeled anti-feminist." He says, "It has nothing to do with being anti-feminist it has to do with speaking the truth about abuse and assault."

Re-thinking the Statute of Limitations and Sensitivity Training

Fradkin and other experts point out that it can take many years for a childhood survivor of sexual abuse to come to terms with what happened to them and finally report it to authorities, even 10 years or more. Many states statute of limitations in bringing charges, however, protect the perpetrators. It is unknown if adult male survivors experience exactly the same difficulties, but it is a good assumption. Certainly, anything police and prosecutors can do to make the process easier for victims should be undertaken. Police, prosecutors, judges, and victim advocates need to become more sensitized to the needs of such victims, and be aware how difficult it is for the male victim to report it. Fradkin says some prosecutors have attended Malesurvivor conferences, but "not enough."

There are rape crisis lines and support centers around the country, but none to his knowledge (or ours) that specialize in helping male victims, though all are there to help female victims and most outreach literature, website information, and other resources are for female victims. In particular, victims' advocates in correction and prosecutor offices need more training in how to help male victims in a more effective manner. Males can be hyper-vigilante about any perceived judgments that may come his way even from a seemingly sympathetic victim advocate, so sensitivity to the particular needs of males, which are mostly similar to female victims of rape and sexual assault, but also different in some ways, is of utmost importance. For example, males may need even more constant reassurance that they had no control over what happened to them—that they did not cause it—it was done to them. They may need to be commended for their courage in coming forward to an even greater extent than female victims as this will reinforce a sense that it is a "manly" thing to do—to confront with courage when an outrage has been perpetrated.

Therapy and the Healing Journey

Fradkin says that when one looks at the resources tab at Malesurvivor. org and seeks a therapist in a particular state, "it looks like a rather paltry list." He says much more needs to be done, particularly in graduate schools where the issue of how to help male victims—whether they are children or adults is not nearly enough a part of the training. 1in6.org, Malesurvivor.org and others do conduct trainings and workshops, but the need is greater than the supply.

Nevertheless, it is of supreme importance that survivors seek help. Fradkin points to these components that make up the healing journey:

1. Recognize that healing is possible. It occurs when men find support in particular from other men. Even in a virtual room, if that is all that is available. It is incredibly helpful and powerful. It will help end isolation and shame.
2. Find a therapist. It is the worst thing in the world to have to educate a therapist about your problem. A therapist should be prepared to work with that particular issue. Ask straightforward specific

questions about their experience and training in helping men with similar issues. "Is this a topic that you have been successful in helping men deal with?"

3. Risk telling someone in their life about what was done. This is part of the healing process of finding support outside of therapy. It is a risk, but a risk that is easier to take when it is recognized that it did not just "happen." Tornadoes and hurricanes "happen." Someone made a choice to do this in an effort to exert power over someone else. That is a choice, not a "happening." The victim is picked because it was perceived by the perpetrator that they were vulnerable, that they could get away with it.

4. Give oneself permission to take time to heal and recover. It will take time. Recognize that a certain level of functionality may not be always able to be maintained and give oneself permission to have those moments. Acknowledge that fear, doubt, shame, frustration are part of what may be experienced and owning these feelings and accepting them as a normal part of what has been experienced is an essential part of the healing process.

5. Offer oneself compassion and forgiveness for what could not be stopped. Recognize that this was an assault. It occurred perhaps because you were vulnerable at the time, but not because you are weak.

The National Center for Victims of Crime offers these further tips for male victims of rape and sexual assault, but we should point out that many, if not most, of this advice (as does the previous advice from Dr. Fradkin) also applies to both genders:

Males also commonly experience many of the reactions that females experience. These reactions include: depression, anger, guilt, self-blame, sexual dysfunctions, flashbacks, and suicidal feelings. Other problems facing males include an increased sense of vulnerability, damaged self-image and emotional distancing. Male rape victims not only have to confront unsympathetic attitudes if they choose to press charges, they also often hear unsupportive statements from their friends, family and acquaintances. People will tend to fault the male victim instead of the rapist. . . .

Research indicates that the most common sites for male rape involving post-puberty victims are outdoors in remote areas and in automobiles (the latter usually involving hitchhikers) . . . Also, multiple sexual acts are more likely to be demanded, weapons are more likely to be displayed and used, and physical injury is more likely to occur, with the injuries that do occur being more serious than with injured female rape victims.

Another major concern facing male rape victims is society's belief that men should be able to protect themselves and, therefore, it is somehow their fault that they were raped. The experience of a rape may affect gay and heterosexual men differently. Most rape counselors point out that gay men have difficulties in their sexual and emotional relationships with other men and think that the assault occurred because they are gay, whereas straight men often begin to question their sexual identity and are more disturbed by the sexual aspect of the assault than the violence involved. . . .

Even if you do not seem injured, it is important to get medical attention. Sometimes injuries that seem minor at first can get worse. Survivors can sometimes contract a sexually transmitted disease during the sexual assault, but not suffer immediate symptoms. Even if the symptoms of that disease take weeks or months to appear, it might be easily treated with an early diagnosis. . . .

Sexual assault and rape are serious crimes. As a sexual assault survivor, you have the right to report the crime to the police. This decision is one *only you* can make. But because authorities are not always sensitive to male sexual assault victims, it is important to have a friend or advocates go with you to report the crime for support and assistance.[59]

If a Tree Falls in the Forest . . .

And no one hears it, does it make a sound? I would argue that it does not, at least in terms of human interaction. The *most* frequent question I am asked on radio talk shows (and this author has done nearly 200 such shows) is: "Aren't Men more reluctant to come forward—because of the fear of ridicule or being called a wimp—to admit abuse at the hands of a woman?"

My answer is always the same. I have talked with as many abused women as I have abused men. I do not know of any of the women who "shouted it from the rooftops" when it was occurring. Many did not tell relatives or closest friends or hid it from them and certainly did not go to the authorities or seek help of any sort until the "last straw." It is the same with men. No more, no less. The difference with men is that no one asks. No one, or very few people, say to them, "I think this is happening to you and maybe you would like to talk about it." Finally, of course, in our media, in our legal system, and elsewhere we have not only no recognition that they exist, but no response, and few or no services for them when they do finally seek help or assistance. They are invisible. And, they remain invisible longer than do women, but only because we *choose* to make them invisible. We make them invisible by denying them services solely because of their sex, and few people, so far at least, have objected to this government, corporate, and non-profit agency sponsored policy. That this policy exists is easily provable for domestic violence approaches. The evidence points to even more severe neglect when it comes to issues of sexual coercion, sexual assault, rape, stalking and sexual harassment.

We can, however, have hope that slowly change is occurring. It must inevitably occur under the realization that the last taboo must be broken. As Dr. Malcolm George pointed out, that last taboo is not really that men can be sexually coerced, sexually assaulted, sexually harassed, raped, and stalked by adult women. The last taboo is that men and women are more alike than they are different.

Notes

Chapter 1

1. Information on the Varga case was obtained via author interviews with prosecutors Jon Love and Patti Connolly-Walker. Connolly-Walker checked a draft copy and verified details with court testimony and prosecutor and police records, 2010.

2. J. Love, interview with author, 2010.

3. P. Overberg, interview with author, 2009.

4. *The Tech*, Massachusetts Institute of Technology, September 24, 1991, http://tech.mit.edu/V110/

5. Alexis Williams, sexual advice columnist, www.thewetspot.com

6. P. Sarrel and W. Masters, "Sexual Molestation of Men by Women," *Archives of Sexual Behavior* 1, no. 2 (1982): 117–131.

7. Ibid., Introduction.

8. U.S. Department of Justice, Bureau of Justice Statistics, *Sex Offenses and Offenders: An Analysis of Data on Rape and Sexual Assault*, February 1997, NCJ-163392, http://bjs.ojp.usdoj.gov/content/pub/pdf/SOO.PDF

9. U.S. Department of Justice, Bureau of Justice Statistics, *Sexual Assault of Young Children as Reported to Law Enforcement*, July 2000, NCJ 182990, http://bjs.ojp.usdoj.gov/content/pub/ascii/saycrle.txt

10. Ibid.

11. U.S. Department of Justice and Centers for Disease Control and Prevention, *Extent, Nature and Consequences of Intimate Partner Violence—Findings from the National Violence Against Women Study*, (2000), NCJ 181867, http://www.cdc.gov/ViolencePrevention/pdf/NISVS_Report2010-a.pdf

12. Ibid.

13. N. W. Pino and R. F. Meier, "Gender Differences in Rape Reporting," *Sex Roles: A Journal of Research* 40, no. 11/12 (1999): 979–990.

14. C. Muehlenhard and S. Cook, "Men's Self Reports of Unwanted Sexual Activity," *Journal of Sex Research* 24, no. 1 (1988): 58–72.

15. J.M. Siegel, S.B. Soreson, J.M. Golding, M.A. Burnam and J.A. Stein, "The Adult Prevalence of Sexual Assault: The Los Angeles Epidemiological Catchment Area Project," *American Journal of Epidemiology* 126, no. 6 (1987): 1154–1164.

16. P.B. Anderson and C.S. Johnson, eds., *Sexually Aggressive Women: Current Perspectives and Controversies* (New York: Garland Publishing, Inc., 1998).

17. Muehlenhard and Cook, "Men's Self Reports."

18. A. Coxell, M. King, G. Mezey and D. Gordon, "Lifetime Prevalence, Characteristics, and Associated Problems of Non-Consensual Sex in Men: Cross Sectional Survey," *British Medical Journal* 318 (1999): 846–50.

19. C.M. Renzetti, *Violent Betrayal: Partner Abuse in Lesbian Relationships* (Beverly Hills, CA: Sage, 1998).

20. Wire reports, *The Oregonian*, March 18, 1998, C4.

21. M.C. Black, K.C. Basile, M.J. Breiding, S.G. Smith, M.L. Walters, M.T. Merrick, J. Chen, and M.R. Stevens, *The National Intimate Partner and Sexual Violence Survey (NISVS): 2010 Summary Report,* National Center for Injury Prevention and Control, Centers for Disease Control and Prevention.

22. Stop Abusive and Violent Environments (SAVE, www.saveservices.org) to the CDC, January 2012.

23. Linda C. DeGutis (DrPH, MSN, Director, National Center for Injury Prevention and Control, CDC), to SAVE, February 1, 2012.

24. SAVE letter to the CDC, January 2012.

25. Ibid.

26. DeGutis to SAVE, February 1, 2012.

27. SAVE to the CDC, January 2012.

28. Ibid.

29. Ibid.

30. Marc Angelucci to the author, email correspondence, December 11, 2011.

31. Howard Fradkin (PhD, director of MaleSurvivor) to the author, email, January 18, 2012.

32. Statement transmitted by email to author, via Howard Fradkin, as a public statement from Ken Followell (President, MaleSurvivor), January 19, 2012.

33. A. Dworkin, *Letters From a War Zone* (New York: Lawrence Hill Books, 1993), 119.

34. C. MacKinnon, *Feminism Unmodified: Discourses on Life and Law* (Harvard, MA: Harvard University Press, 1988), 82.

35. Ibid, 88.

36. Think Tank Transcripts, "A Conversation with Catharine MacKinnon," July 7, 1995, http://www.pbs.org/thinktank/transcript215.html

37. C. Paglia, *Vamps and Tramps* (New York: Vintage Books, 1994), 24–25.

38. Email correspondence with author, December 11, 2011.

39. Feminist Majority Foundation, "Feminist Majority Foundation Celebrates FBI Approval of New Rape Definition," January 6, 2012, http://feminist.org/news/pressstory.asp?id=13402

40. "We did it! FBI Director Robert Mueller Approved the Change Recommended by Several Committees of the FBI's Criminal Justice Information Service to update the FBI Uniform Crime Report definition of rape!," http://feminist.org/nomoreexcuses/rapeisrape.asp

41. "What Is Consent?" Vassar Sexual Assault Violence Prevention, http://savp.vassar.edu/facts/consent.html

42. http://www.loveologyuniversity.com/DrAvaPages/Sexual_Consent_Form.html#. Note: The form itself can be found here: http://www.loveologyuniversity.com/Images/DrAvaResourceFile/Resource_168_Sexual_Consent_Form.pdf

43. C. Paglia, *Vamps and Tramps*, 25–26.

44. National Center For Victims of Crime, http://www.ncvc.org/ncvc/main.aspx?dbName=DocumentViewer&DocumentID=32361

45. Ibid.

46. W. Kierski, "Female Violence: Can We Therapists Face Up to It?" *Counselling and Psychotherapy Journal* 13, no. 10 (2002): 32–35.

47. M. Petrovich and D. Templar, "Heterosexual Molestation of Children Who Later Become Rapists," *Psychological Reports* 54 (1984): 810.

48. "Can Women Rape Men?" Feminist Critics (blog), January 5, 2009, http://www.feministcritics.org/blog/2009/01/05/can-women-rape-men-rp/

49. Sexual Violence National Center For Victims of Crime, http://www.victimsofcrime.org

50. P. J. Isely and D. Gehrenbeck-Shim, "Sexual Assault of Men in the Community," *Journal of Community Psychology* 25, no. 2 (1997): 159–166.

51. "The Helpseeking Experiences of Men Who Sustain Intimate Partner Violence: An Overlooked Population and Implications for Practice," http://www.clarku.edu/faculty/dhines/Douglas%20%20Hines%202011%20helpseeking%20experiences%20of%20male%20victims.pdf

52. M. Famworth and R. Teske, "Gender Differences in Felony Court Processing, *Women in Criminal Justice* 6, no. 2 (1995): 23–44.

53. C. Spohn and D. Bichner, "Is Preferential Treatment of Female Offenders a Thing of the Past? A Multisite Study of Gender Race and Imprisonment," *Criminal Justice Policy Review* 11, no. 2 (2000): 149–184.

54. R. Embry and P. Lyons Jr., "Sex-Based Sentencing Discrepancies between Male and Female Sex Offenders," *Feminist Criminology* 7, no. 2 (2012): 146–162.

55. "Woman Jailed for Testicle Attack," BBC News, February 10, 2005, http://news.bbc.co.uk/2/hi/4253849.stm

56. *Willan v. Willan*, 2 All. E.R. 463 (CA 1960) at 466. Quoted from Aimee L. Widor, "Comment: Fact or Fiction?: Role-Reversal Sexual Harassment in the Modern Workplace," *University of Pittsburgh Law Review* 58 (1996): 225, 232. See also http://www.malesurvivor.org/Reversal_of_Fortune.pdf

57. W. Storr, "The Rape of Men," http://www.guardian.co.uk/society/2011/jul/17/the-rape-of-men

Chapter 2

1. Alex Kuczynski, "She's Got to Be a Macho Girl—In a Role Reversal, Teenage Girls Are the Aggressors When It Comes to Boys," *The New York Times*, November 3, 2002, section 9, p. 1.

2. "Coercion," http://www.answers.com/topic/coercion/

3. "Coercion," *Stanford Encyclopedia of Philosophy*, http://plato.stanford.edu/entries/coercion/

4. "Coercion," http://www.newworldencyclopedia.org/entry/Coercion/

5. Ibid.

6. M.C. Black, K.C. Basile, M.J. Breiding, S.G. Smith, M.L. Walters, M.T. Merrick, J. Chen and M.R. Stevens, *The National Intimate Partner and Sexual Violence Survey (NISVS): 2010 Summary Report,* Atlanta, GA: National Center for Injury Prevention and Control, Centers for Disease Control and Prevention, 2011.

7. Kuczynski, "She's Got to Be a Macho Girl."

8. National Coalition for Men, http://ncfm.org/2011/03/news/dating-abuse/, September, 2011.

9. David Hemenway, Deborah Prothrow-Stith and Angela Browne, "Report of the 2004 Boston Youth Survey," August 2005, Boston, 1–114, http://www.hsph.harvard.edu/hyvpc/files/2004BYSfullreport.pdf/

10. Centers for Disease Control and Prevention, "Youth Risk Behavior Surveillance-United States, 2005," http://www.cdc.gov/mmwr/pdf/ss/ss5505.pdf/

11. Martin S. Fiebert, "References Examining Assaults by Women on Their Spouses or Male Partners: An Annotated Bibliography," May 2011, Long Beach, http://www.csulb.edu/~mfiebert/assault.htm

12. Martin S. Fiebert, "References Examining Men as Victims of Women's Sexual Coercion," http://www.dottal.org/LBDUK/references_examining_men_as_vict.htm/

13. News Release, University of Washington, "College Men Nearly as Likely as Women to Report They Are Victims of Unwanted Sexual Coercion," http://www.fact.on.ca/newpaper/wa990726.htm

14. C.C. Cochran, P.A. Frazier, A.M. Olson, "Predictors of Responses to Unwanted Sexual Attention," *Psychology of Women Quarterly* 21 (1997): 207–226.

15. M.A. Straus, S.L. Hamby, S. Boney-McCoy and D.G. Sugarman, "Development and Preliminary Psychometric Data," *Journal of Family Issues* 17 (1996): 283–315.

16. J.L. Baier, M.G. Rosenzweig and E.G. Whipple, "Patterns of Sexual Behavior, Coercion and Victimization of University Students," *Journal of College Student Development* 32 (1991): 310–322.

17. L.K. Waldner-Haugrud and B. Magruder, "Male and Female Sexual Victimization in Dating Relationships. Gender Differences in Coercion Techniques and Outcomes," *Violence and Victims* 10 (1995): 203–215.

18. J.L. Carr, *American College Health Association Campus Violence white paper*, 2005, Baltimore, MD: http://wellness.buffalo.edu/wes/whitepaper.pdf

19. I.L. Lottes and M.S. Weinberg, "Sexual Coercion among University Students: A Comparison of the United States and Sweden," *Journal of Sex Research* 34 (1996): 67–76.

20. P.I. Erickson, D.P.H. Rapkin and A.J. Rapkin, "Unwanted Sexual Experiences among Middle and High School Youth," *Journal of Adolescent Health* 12 (1991): 319–325.

21. L.P. Rouse, "Abuse in Dating Relationships: A Comparison of Blacks, Whites, and Hispanics," *Journal of College Student Development* 29 (1988): 312–319.

22. L. Garcia, L. Milano and A. Quijano, "Perceptions of Coercive Sexual Behavior by Males and Females," *Sex Roles* 21 (1989): 569–577.

23. L. Margolin, "Gender and the Stolen Kiss: The Social Support of Male and Female to a Violent Partner's Sexual Consent in a Noncoercive Situation," *Archives of Sexual Behavior* 19 (1990): 281–291.

24. C.L. Muehlenhard and S.W. Cook, "Men's Self Reports of Unwanted Sexual Activity," *The Journal of Sex Research* 24 (1998): 58–72.

25. R.E. Smith, C.J. Pine, and M.E. Hawley, "Social Cognitions About Adult Male Victims of Female Sexual Assault," *Journal of Sex Research* 24 (1988): 101–112.

26. C. Struckman-Johnson and D. Struckman-Johnson, "College Men and Women's Reactions to Hypothetical Sexual Touch Varied by Initiator Gender and Coercion Level," *Sex Roles* 29 (1993): 371–385.

27. C.J. Struckman-Johnson, D.L. Struckman-Johnson, and P.B. Anderson, "Tactics of Sexual Coercion: When Men and Women Won't Take No for an Answer," *Journal of Sex Research* 40 (1) (2003): 76–86.

28. Donna Laframboise, "Unwanted Advances: New Research from the University of Guelph Concludes That the Role of Sexual Predator Is No Longer the Domain of Men," http://www.fact.on.ca/newpaper/np98120d.htm

29. M.C. Black, K.C. Basile, M.J. Breiding, S.G. Smith, M.L. Walters, M.T. Merrick, J. Chen, and M.R. Stevens, *The National Intimate Partner and Sexual Violence Survey (NISVS): 2010 Summary Report*, National Center for Injury Prevention and Control, Centers for Disease Control and Prevention, http://www.cdc.gov/ViolencePrevention/pdf/NISVS_Report2010-a.pdf

30. Bert H. Hoff, "National Study: More Men than Women Victims of Intimate Partner Physical Violence, Psychological Aggression. Over 40% of Victims of Severe Physical Violence are Men," MenWeb (2012): http://www.batteredmen.com/NISVS.htm (ISSN: 1095–5240 http://www.batteredmen.com/NISVS.htm), used by permission.

31. *Los Angeles Times*, http://latimesblogs.latimes.com/lanow/2011/07/orange-county-prosecutors-charged-a-garden-grove-woman-wednesday-with-two-felony-counts-for-allegedly-cutting-off-her-husband.html

32. S. A. Hughes, "The Talk Ladies Under Fire for Laughing at Catherine Kieu Story," http://www.washingtonpost.com/blogs/celebritology/post/the-talk-ladies-under-fire-for-laughing-at-catherine-kieu-story-video/2011/07/18/gIQA3OjkLI_blog.html

33. The Talk Weekdays, "The Talk Video—The Talk—12/23/2011." CBS.com. http://www.cbs.com/daytime/the_talk/video/?pid=ta8Q6UydH70mtlwj2JMmKc1jHAnmyjcq&vs=Full%20Episodes&play=true/

34. Patricia Tjaden and Nancy Thoennes, *Prevalence, Incidence, and Consequences of Violence Against Women: Findings from the National Violence Against Women Survey*, National Institute of Justice, Centers for Disease Control and Prevention, (1998), https://www.ncjrs.gov/pdffiles/172837.pdf

35. L. A. Johnson, "A Model Treatment Program for Incarcerated Female Sex Offenders" (PhD diss., Carlos Albizu University, 2002), *Dissertation Abstracts International 63* (2002): 4906.

36. The Criminal Code of Canada, http://www.sacc.to/sya/crime/law.htm

37. "Was I Raped?" Rape, Abuse & Incest National Network, http://www.rainn.org/get-information/types-of-sexual-assault/was-it-rape, January 2010.

38. The National Center for Victims of Crime, "Sexual Assault," http://www.ncvc.org/ncvc/main.aspx?dbName=DocumentViewer&DocumentID=32369#1

39. Sexual Abuse, Title 18, Chapter 109A, Sections 2241–2233.

40. D. C. Weiss, "School Backs Off Claim that Playground Touching by 6-Year-Old Was Sexual Assault," ABA Journal website, January 30, 2012, http://www.abajournal.com/news/article/school_backs_off_claim_that_playground_touching_by_6-year-old_was_sexual_as/

41. G. Ahuja, "First-Grader Suspended for Sexual Harassment,"*ABC News*, February 7, 2006, http://abcnews.go.com/US/story?id=1591633

42. C. Broderick, "Prosecutor of Bottom-Swatting Boys is Arrested in Alleged Assault," *The Oregonian*-Oregonlive: December 18, 2008, http://www.oregonlive.com/news/index.ssf/2008/12/prosecutor_of_buttswatting_boy.html

43. Weiss, "School Backs Off."

44. M. C. Black, K. C. Basile, M. J. Breiding, S. G. Smith, M. L. Walters, M. T. Merrick, J. Chen and M. R. Stevens, *The National Intimate Partner and Sexual Violence Survey (NISVS): 2010 Summary Report,* National Center for Injury Prevention and Control, Centers for Disease Control and Prevention, http://www.cdc.gov/ViolencePrevention/pdf/NISVS_Report2010-a.pdf

45. Ibid., 18–19.

46. Ibid., 19.

47. Bureau of Justice Statistics, "One in 34 U.S. Adults Under Correctional Supervision in 2011, Lowest Rate Since 2000," http://www.bjs.gov/content/pub/press/cpus11ppus11pr.cfm

48. M. C. Black et al., 18–19.

49. Ibid., 48.

50. B. H. Hoff, *National Study*.

51. U.S. Department of Justice, Office of Justice Programs, *Survey of State Prison Inmates, 1991: Women in Prison*, Bureau of Justice Statistics Special Report NCJ-145321 (Washington, DC: Government Printing Office, 1994), 4.

52. Fox Butterfield, "Women Find a New Arena for Equality: Prison," *The New York Times*, December 29, 2003.

53. R. Miller, "Hammer Blows, Stabbing with Scissors Helped Cause Boy-friend's Kidney Failure," *The Express-Times*, www.nj.com. May 20, 1994.

54. Associated Press, Saint Louis, Missouri, March 6, 2003.

55. Kim Bell, "Sex Crimes by Women Drawing More Notice," *Saint Louis Post-Dispatch*, March 24, 2003.

56. E.S. Byers, "How Well Does the Traditional Sexual Script Explain Sexual Coercion? Review of a Program of Research," in E. S. Byers and L. F. O'Sullivan, eds., *Sexual Coercion in Dating Relationships* (New York: Haworth Press, 1996), 7–25.

57. Reuters Health; Adrian Coxell, Michael King, Gillian Mezey and Dawn Gordon, "Lifetime Prevalence, Characteristics, and Associated Problems of Non-Consensual Sex in Men: Cross Sectional Survey," *British Medical Journal* 318 (March 27, 1999): 846–850. DOI: 10.1136/bmj.318.7187.846

58. Malcolm George, MD, private paper prepared for this book, email sent on March 6, 1998. Used by permission.

59. Ibid.; P.M. Sarrel and W.H. Masters, "Sexual Molestation of Men by Women," *Archives of Sexual Behavior* 11 (1982): 117–131.

60. C. Struckman-Johnson, "Forced Sex on Dates: It Can Happen to Men, Too," *The Journal of Sex Research* 24 (1988): 58–72.

61. Muehlenhard and Cook, "Men's Self Reports."

62. M.J. George, "Riding the Donkey Backwards: Men as the Unacceptable Victims of Marital Violence," *Journal of Men's Studies* 3, no. 2 (1994): 137–159.

63. C.K. Waterman, L.T. Dawson and J.J. Bogna, "Sexual Coercion in Gay Male and Lesbian Relationships: Predicators and Implications for Support Services," *Journal of Sex Research* 26 (1989):118–124.

64. C.M. Renzettic, *Violent Betrayal: Partner Abuse in Lesbian Relationships* (Beverly Hills, CA: Sage, 1992).

Chapter 3

1. I. Berkow, *Baseball Natural: The Story of Eddie Waitkus* (Carbondale and Edwardsville, IL: Southern Illinois University Press, 2002).

2. Mike Celizic, "Celebrity Stalkers Pose Real Threat to Famous," May 2008, http://today.msnbc.msn.com/id/24425310/ns/today-entertainment/t/celebrity-stalkers-pose-real-threat-famous/

3. P. Tjaden, and N. Thoennes, *Stalking in America: Findings from the National Violence Against Women Survey* (Denver, CO: Center for Policy Research, 1997).

4. P. Tjaden and N. Thoennes, *Stalking in America: Findings from the National Violence Against Women Survey* (U.S. Department of Justice, Office of Justice Programs, National Institute of Justice, April 1998).

5. The National Center for Victims of Crime/Stalking, http://www.ncvc.org/

6. Paul E. Mullen, Michele Pathé, Rosemary Purcell and Geoffrey W. Stuart, "Study of Stalkers," *American Journal of Psychiatry* 156 (1999): 1244–1249.

7. J.R. Meloy, K. Mohandie and M. Green, "The Female Stalker," *Behavioral Sciences & the Law* 29 (2) (2011): 240–54, http://www.ncbi.nlm.nih.gov/pubmed/21351135/

8. P. Mullen, M. Pathé, R. Purcell, *Stalkers and Their Victims* (London: Cambridge University Press, 2000).

9. Tara Palmatier, "Female Stalkers, Part 1: What Is Stalking and Can Men Be Stalked by Women?" *Shrink4Men blog*, February 8, 2011, http://www.shrink4men.com/2011/02/08/stalking-part-i-what-is-stalking-and-can-men-be-stalked-by-women

10. P. Tjaden, *Stalking in America*.

11. Supplemental Victimization Survey (SVS-1), U.S. Department of Justice, http://bjs.ojp.usdoj.gov/content/pub/pdf/svs1_06.pdf/

12. K.E. Davis, A.L. Coker and M. Sanderson, "Physical and Mental Health Effects of Being Stalked for Men and Women," *Violence and Victims* 4 (August 17, 2002): 429–43.

13. Rita Handrich, "Women Who Stalk: Who They Are and How They Do It," http://keenetrial.com/blog/2011/06/01/women-who-stalk-who-they-are-and-how-they-do-it/

14. Sara G. West and Susan Hatters Friedman, MD, "These Boots Are Made for Stalking: Characteristics of Female Stalkers," http://www.innovationscns.com/these-boots-are-made-for-stalking-characteristics-of-female-stalkers/

15. Katrina Baum, Shannan Catalano, Michael Rand and Kristina Rose, "Stalking Victimization in the United States," *National Crime Victimization Survey*, January 2009, http://www.ncvc.org/src/AGP.Net/Components/DocumentViewer/Download.aspxnz?DocumentID=45862

16. Susan Carroll, "1,001 Phone Calls, Tire Irons, Sword and Eggs," *San Antonio Express News*, October 13, 2011, 5B.

17. Ibid.

18. "Woman Guilty of Stalking Doctor—A Woman Who Terrorised a Psychiatrist and His Fiancee for Three Years Is Warned She May Face a Long Jail Term," http://news.bbc.co.uk/go/em/fr/-/2/hi/uk_news/england/london/5239656.stm/

19. J. Reid Meloy and Cynthia Boyd, "Female Stalkers and Their Victims," *The Journal of the American Academy of Psychiatry and the Law* 31 (2003): 211–219, http://www.ncfm.org/libraryfiles/Children/women%20behave%20bad/Female%20stalkers.pdf/

20. R. Purcell, M. Pathé and P. Mullen, "A Study of Women Who Stalk," *American Journal of Psychiatry* 158, no. 12 (2001): 2056–60.

21. Ibid.

22. Michael G. Conner, "Stalking: Why Do Men and Women Stalk Each Other?" http://www.crisiscounseling.com/articles/stalking.htm/

23. U.S. Department of Justice, Tjaden and Thoennes, *Prevalence, Incidence, and Consequence*.

24. Charles Corry, "Stalking Defined by Charles E. Corry, Ph.D.," Domestic Violence against Men in Colorado website, last modified November 14, 2012, http://www.dvmen.org/dv-41.htm

25. Tara Palmatier, "Female Stalkers, Part 4: Attachment Style as a Predictor of Who Is More Likely to Stalk and Abuse and Who Is More Likely to Be Stalked and Abused," February 8, 2011, http://www.shrink4men.com/2011/02/

26. Helen Pidd, "Cyberstalking: Tackling the 'Faceless Cowards'," *The Guardian*, September 23, 2010, http://www.guardian.co.uk/uk/2010/sep/24/ukcrime-police/

27. Ariel (Penn State), "Facebook Creepin—A Guide," August 3, 2010, http://collegecandy.com/2010/08/03/facebook-creepin-a-guide/

28. Carsten Maple, Emma Short and Antony Brown, *Cyberstalking in the United Kingdom: An Analysis of the ECHO Pilot Survey*, 2011, University of Bedfordshire, http://www.beds.ac.uk/__data/assets/pdf_file/0003/83109/Final_Report.pdf/

29. Daily Mail Reporter, "How Facebook is Turning Women into Stalkers: A Third of Online Victims Are Now Men," *The Daily Mail*, http://www.dailymail.co.uk/sciencetech/article-1365529/How-Facebook-turning-women-stalkers-A-online-victims-men.html#ixzz1cDxQYxzP/

30. SPAMfighter News, "More Men Fall Victim to Cyber Stalking than Women," September 26, 2007, http://www.spamfighter.com/News-9105-More-Men-fall-Victims-to-Cyber-Stalking-than-Women.htm/. See also: Ian Williams, "Men More Likely to be Cyber-Stalking Victims," V3.co.uk website, September 11, 2007, http://www.v3.co.uk/v3-uk/news/1940758/men-cyber-stalking-victims/; Stefan Fafinski and Neshan Minassian, *UK CyberCrime Report 2009*, Invenio Research, http://www.garlik.com/file/cybercrime_report_attachement/

31. Colleen O'Brien, "NW Woman Editor Charged with Identity Theft, Cyberstalking," KXLY, July 12, 2011, http://www.kxly.com/news/28527467/detail.html/

32. Meloy and Boyd, "Female Stalkers."

33. Doris Hall, "Outside Looking In: Stalkers and Their Victims," California State University-Bakersfield, www.csub.edu/~dhall/crju430/Outside_Looking_In.ppt

34. Mullen, *Stalkers and Their Victims*.

35. C. Kuehner, P. Gass, H. Dressing, "Mediating Effects of Stalking Victimization on Gender Differences in Mental Health," *Journal of Interpersonal Violence* 27, no. 2 (January 2012): 199–221.

36. Sheryl Pimlott-Kubiak and Lilia M. Cortina, "Gender, Victimization, and Outcomes: Reconceptualizing Risk," *Journal of Consulting and Clinical Psychology* 71, no. 3 (2003): 528–539.

37. The National Center for Victims of Crime, http://www.victimsofcrime.org/our-programs/stalking-resource-center/help-for-victims/

38. Note: At the time of completing the notes, www.survivorsinaction.org appears to have removed this letter from their website. However, we did find this statement: "In 2013 tragically victims continue to reach out to the above listed agencies and others at the state and local level that are funded, only to discover that they are referred, ignored or denied needed support services." The NNEDV was one of the listed agencies.

39. Note: The Stalking Resource Center website describes themselves: "In 2000, the National Center for Victims of Crime partnered with the U.S. Department of Justice Office on Violence Against Women to create the Stalking Resource Center (SRC)," http://www.victimsofcrime.org/our-programs/stalking-resource-center/about-us.Note: Information on the planned conference is no longer listed on the website.

40. Note: The Survivors in Action website no longer gives the full text of this post. It was retrieved in July of 2012. www.survivorsinaction.org. However, other similar letters by the group (not affiliated with SAVE) can be found at: www.saveservices.org

41. P. Cook, *Abused Men: The Hidden Side of Domestic Violence* (Santa Barbara, CA: Praeger/ABC-Clio, 2009), 124.

Chapter 4

1. K. Velie, and D. Blackburn, "Police Chief Accused of Sexually Assaulting Her Officers," Cal Coast News, January 26, 2012, http://calcoastnews.com/2012/01/police-chief-accused-of-sexually-assaulting-her-officers/

2. A. Rodrigue, "Assistant Police Chief under Investigation for Sexual harassment," WBRZ TV, October 25, 2011, http://www.wbrz.com/news/zachary-assistant-police-chief-under-investigation-for-sexual-harassment/

3. "Mountainburg Police Chief Accused of Sexual Harrasment," KFSM/KXNW, http://www.5newsonline.com/news/rivervalley/kfsm-mountainburg-police-chief-accused-of-sexual-harassment-20110908,0,4310700.story

4. J. Mundy, "Sexual Harassment amongst Officers—California Labor Law Violation," Lawyers and Settlements.com, http://www.lawyersandsettlements.com/articles/california_labor_law/california-labor-law-lawsuit-11–17671.html

5. P. Bentley, "Lesbian PSCO 'Fondled Colleagues Breasts and Groped Male Officers during String of Sexual Assaults'," *The Daily Mail,* May 9, 2012, http://www.dailymail.co.uk/news/article-2141849/Female-PCSO-fondled-colleagues-breasts-string-sexual-assaults-fellow-officers.html#ixzz21xGTC0Ko

6. Hearings before the Committee on the Judiciary: Hearing on the Nomination of Clarence Thomas to be Associate Justice of the Supreme Court of the United States, Day 1, Session 1, 102nd Cong.

7. Policy Guidance on Current Issues of Sexual Harassment, EEOC, § 1604.11.

8. *Robinson v. Jacksonville Shipyards,* 760 F. Supp. 1486 (1991), 57 FEP Cases 971 (M.D. Fla.).

9. I. H. Settles, Z.A.T. Harrell, N.T. Buchanon and S.C.Y. Yap, "Frightened or Bothered: Two Types of Sexual Harassment Appraisals," *Social Psychological and Personality Science* 2, no. 6 (2011): 600-608, as discussed in "Study Finds Surprising Gender Differences Related to Sexual Harassment," *ScienceDaily,* April 1, 2011, http://www.sciencedaily.com/releases/2011/03/110330101242.htm

10. *Sexual Harassment in the Federal Workplace: Trends, Progress and Continuing Challenges,* A Report to the President and the Congress of the United States, Washington, D.C., USMSPB. 1995, U.S. Merit Systems Protection Board.

11. Equal Employment Opportunity Commission, National Data Base, http://www.eeoc.gov/eeoc/statistics/enforcement/sexual_harassment.cfm

12. Marie Price, "EEOC: More Men Filing Complaints of Sexual Harassment," *The Oklahoma City Journal Record*, August 22, 2008, Oklahoma City.

13. Ibid.

14. "Sexual Harassment Charges: EEOC & FEPAs Combined: FY 1997-FY 2011," U.S. Equal Employment Opportunity Commission, http://www.eeoc.gov/eeoc/statistics/enforcement/sexual_harassment.cfm

15. Catherine Hill and Elena Silva, *Drawing the Line: Sexual Harassment on Campus* (Washington, D.C.: American Association of University Women Educational Foundation, 2005): 14, http://www.aauw.org/resource/drawing-the-line-sexual-harassment-on-campus/

16. "Take Back the Campus! Take Back the Radical Feminist Assault on Truth," Independent Women's Forum, http://iwf.org/files/6419ffcf970e1ee07c551a6801c49f25.pdf

17. S. Welsh, "Gender and Sexual Harassment," *Annual Review of Sociology* 25 (1999): 175.

18. "Facts about Sexual Harassment," U.S. Equal Employment Opportunity Commission (EEOC), http://www.eeoc.gov/eeoc/publications/fs-sex.cfm

19. United States Court of Appeals, Seventh Circuit, *Doe v. City of Belleville*, Illinois, 119 F.3b 563 (7th Cir. 1997), http://caselaw.findlaw.com/us-7th-circuit/1297377.html

20. "Facts about Sexual Harassment," U.S. EEOC.

21. Welsh, "Gender," 170.

22. "Facts about Sexual Harassment," U.S. EEOC.

23. Kaushik Basu, "The Economics and Law of Sexual Harassment in the Workplace," *The Journal of Economic Perspectives* 17, no. 3 (2003): 143.

24. Associated Press, "Chain Must Pay Male Sex-Harassment Victim," *The New York Times*, November 24, 1995, http://www.nytimes.com/1995/11/24/us/chain-must-pay-malesex-harassment-victim.html

25. Eve Tahmincioglu, "Male Sexual Harassment Is Not a Joke: It's Real and Reported Cases Are on the Rise—Here's How to Handle It," MSNBC, July 10, 2007, http://www.msnbc.msn.com/id/19536167/ns/business-careers/t/male-sexual-harassment-not-joke

26. Anna North, "She Would Caress His Shoulders and Neck: Female Sexual Harassment Gets Its Moment," *Jezebel,* March 4, 2010, http://jezebel.com/5485603/she-would-caress-his-shoulders-and-neck-female-sexual-harassment-gets-its-moment.

27. Ibid.

28. A. E. Street, J.L. Gradus, J. Stafford and K. Kelly, "Gender Differences in Experiences of Sexual Harassment: Data from a Male-Dominated Environment," *Journal of Consulting Clinical Psychology* 75, no. 3 (2007): 464.

29. Richard Hall, *Sociology of Work Perspectives, Analyses, and Issues* (N.P.: The Pine Forge Press Social Science Library, 1997).

30. Ibid.

31. "Sexual Harassment in the Workplace When the Victim Is Male," http://www.sanfrancisco-employment-lawyer.com/2010/11/sexual-harassment-in-the-workplace-when-the-victim-is-male.shtml. Note: This website appears to be no longer active, the article was retrieved in October, 2011.

32. Alliance Training and Consulting, http://www.alliancetac.com/

33. Speakers Bureau & Workshop Training, http://www.9to5.org/resources/trainings.

34. Diversity in the Workplace—Building a Work Environment Where Performance Thrives, http://www.diversitybuilder.com/diversity_training.php

35. W. Farrell, *The Myth of Male Power* (New York: Simon and Schuster, 1993), 300.

36. Ibid., 307.

37. Ibid., 293.

38. Daphne Patai, *Heterophobia: Sexual Harassment and the Future of Feminism* (Lanham, MD: Rowman & Littlefield, 1998), Preface, xii.

39. Wendy McElroy, "Sexual Harassment ... and Beyond," Speech in Las Vegas, Nevada, May 4, 2002, FEE National Convention.

40. Patai, *Heterophobia*, Preface, xv.

41. E. F. Paul, "Bare Buttocks and Federal Cases," *Society* 35, no. 2 (Jan/Feb 1998): 352–355.

42. Joan Kennedy Taylor, "America's Overproductive Sexual Harassment Law," Cato Institute website, http://www.cato.org/pub_display.php?pub_id=4735. This article first appeared in *Investor's Business Daily*, April 6, 2000.

43. Basu, 154.

Chapter 5

1. Ron Still, former police chief, Portland, Oregon, in a pre-publication review comment for *Abused Men: The Hidden Side of Domestic Violence*, P. W. Cook (Westport, CT: Greenwood/Praeger, 1997).

2. L. Menand, "The War of All Against All," *The New Yorker*, March 14, 1994, 85.

3. Philip Cook, "Men Should Be More than a National Afterthought," OregonLive.com, June 1, 2010, http://www.oregonlive.com/opinion/index.ssf/2010/06/men_should_be_more_than_a_nati.html/

4. Farrell, *Myth of Male Power*, 105.

5. C. Struckman-Johnson, "Forced Sex on Dates: It Can Happen to Men, Too," *The Journal of Sex Research* 24 (1988): 58–72.

6. Note: More information about the survey findings can be found at http://www.saveservices.org/falsely-accused/survey/results

7. Nico Trocme and Nicholas Bala, "False Allegations of Abuse and Neglect When Parents Separate," *Child Abuse and Neglect* 29 (2005): Table 3.

8. Eugene Kanin, "False Rape Allegations," *Archives of Sexual Behavior* 23, no. 1 (1994): 81–92.

9. Ibid.

10. Charles McDowell, "False Allegations," *Forensic Science* 11, no. 4 (1985).

11. Innocence Project, http://www.innocenceproject.org/Content/How_many_people_have_been_exonerated_through_DNA_testing.php/

12. Kimberly Lonsway, Joanne Archambault and David Lisak, "False Reports: Moving Beyond the Issue to Successfully Investigate and Prosecute Non-Stranger Sexual Assault," *The National Center for the Prosecution of Violence Against Women,* http://www.ndaa.org/pdf/the_voice_vol_3_no_1_2009.pdf/

13. S. R. Gross, "How Many False Convictions Are There? How Many Exonerations Are There?" in *Wrongful Convictions and Miscarriages of Justice: Causes and Remedies in North American and European Criminal Justice Systems,* ed. C.R. Huff and M. Killias (Routledge, 2013, University of Michigan Public Law Research Paper No. 316).

14. Ula Ilnytzky, "NYPD Boss' Son Returns to TV Show After Rape Claim," Associated Press, February 10, 2012.

15. Colleen Long, "NYPD Boss' Son, Not Charged, Returns to TV Friday," Associated Press, February 8, 2012.

16. National Registry of Exonerations, http://www.law.umich.edu/special/exoneration/Pages/detaillist.aspx

17. "Crossing the Line: Responding to Prosecutorial Misconduct," ABA Section of Litigation Annual Conference, April 16–18, 2008. See also, National Association of Criminal Defense Lawyers, http://www.nacdl.org/default.aspx

18. Zack Hudson, "Jury Acquits Rucker Smith," *Americus Times-Recorder,* May 5, 2006, http://www.americustimesrecorder.com/siteSearch/apstorysection/local_story_125003348.html/

19. E. Epstein, "Speaking the Unspeakable," *Massachusetts Bar Association Newsletter,* 1993.

20. Katie Roiphe, *The Morning After: Sex, Fear and Feminism on Campus* (New York: Little, Brown, 1993).

21. Nara Schoenberg and Sam Roe, "The Making of an Epidemic," *Toledo Blade,* October 10, 1993; Neil Gilbert, "Examining the Facts: Advocacy Research Overstates the Incidence of Data and Acquaintance Rape," in *Current Controversies in Family Violence,* ed. Richard Gelles and Donileen Loseke (Newbury Park, CA: Sage Publications, 1993), 120–132; Campus Crime and Security, Washington, D.C.: U.S. Department of Education, 1997. According to this study, campus police reported 1,310 forcible sex offenses on U.S. campuses in one year. That works out to an average of fewer than one rape per campus. See also "The False Rape Society: Community of the Wrongly Accused, http://falserapesociety.blogspot.com/2011/10/men-of-brown-university-your-school.html/

22. Heather Mac Donald, "The Campus Rape Myth," *City Journal* 18, no. 1 (Winter 2008), http://www.city-journal.org/2008/18_1_campus_rape.html./

23. Ibid.

24. S. Hingston, "The New Rules of College Sex: How the Federal Government and a Malvern Lawyer are Rewriting the Rules on Campus Hookups—and Tagging Young Men as Dangerous Predators," *Philadelphia Magazine*, September 2011, http://www.phillymag.com/articles/the-new-rules-of-college-sex/

25. H. Mac Donald, "The Campus Rape Myth," *City Journal* 18, no. 1 (Winter 2008), http//'www.city-journal.org/2008_1_campus_rape.html/

26. Ibid.

27. "Victory for Due Process: Student Punished for Alleged Sexual Assault Cleared by University of North Dakota; Accuser Still Wanted for Lying to Police," *FIRE Defending Individual Rights in Higher Education*, October 18, 2011, http://thefire.org/article/13758.html

28. H. Mac Donald, "The Campus Rape Myth."

29. Ibid.

30. Hingston, "The New Rules of College Sex."

31. "Sex Smears and the Rule of Law at Yale," *Wall Street Journal*, February 4, 2012, http://online.wsj.com/public/search?article-doc-type=%7BCommentary+%28U.S.%29%7D&HEADER_TEXT=commentary+%28u.s/

32. Philip Cook and Glenn Sacks, "The Mysterious Decline of Men on Campus," in *Abuse Your Illusions,* ed. R. Kick (New York: Disinformation Press, 2003), 77–81.

33. Mark Perry, "Huge College Degree Gap for Class of 2010," *Carpe Diem* blog, May 11, 2010, http://mjperry.blogspot.com/2010/05/huge-college-degree-gap-for-class-of.html/

34. Christine Stolba, "Lying in a Room of One's Own: How Women's Studies Textbooks Miseducate Students," Independent Women's Forum white paper, 2002, 31–32.

35. Ibid.

36. Ibid., 19.

37. Ibid., 23.

38. "Take Back the Campus," *Daily Bruin*, April 18, 2001.

39. Leo, "Miffing the Myth Makers: A Feisty Student Newspaper Ad Roils the College Feminists," *Jewish World Review.com*, May 31, 2001.

40. Barrie Levy, "Bruin Ad Misleading," *Daily Bruin*, May 5, 2001.

41. Mason Stockstill, "Students Protest Publication of Ad in Newspaper," *Daily Bruin*, May 5, 2001.

42. Leo, "Miffing the myth markers."

43. Christina Hoff Sommers, *The War Against Boys: How Misguided Feminism is Harming Our Young Men* (New York: Simon & Schuster, 2000), 161–64.

44. Ibid., 162.

45. Simon Fraser Student Society, Women's Centre, http://www.sfuwomenctr.ca/faqs.html/

46. R. Urback, "Robin Urback on Shocking Anti-Male Hatred on the Simon Fraser University Campus," *The National Post,* December, 2000, http://full comment.nationalpost.com/2012/05/20/robyn-urback-on-shocking-anti-male-hatred-on-the-sfu-campus/

47. Cook and Sacks, "The Mysterious Decline of Men on Campus."

48. Farrell, *Myth of Male Power,* 307–8.

49. Nordstrom, Corporate Governance, Code of Business Conduct and Ethics, November 17, 2010, http://phx.corporate-ir.net/phoenix.zhtml?c=93295&p=irol-govConduct/

50. Mauricio Velasquez, "A New Era in Sexual Harassment," Sexual Harassment Prevention Center, http://stopharass.com/article-sexual-harassment.htm/

51. James Taranto, "Sexual Harassment Stories: A Report from the Field Illustrates Both the Need and Danger of Regulations," November 2011, *Wall Street Journal* online, November 2011, http://online.wsj.com/article/SB100014240 52970203804204577017862365156578.html?fb_ref=wsj_share_FB&fb_source=home_oneline/

52. Ibid.

53. L.P. Sheridan and E. Blaauw, "Characteristics of False Stalking Reports," *Criminal Justice and Behavior* 31, no. 1 (2004): 55–72. "After eight uncertain cases were excluded, the false reporting rate was judged to be 11.5%, with the majority of false victims suffering delusions (70%)."

54. Seth Brown, "Reality of Persecutory Beliefs: Base Rate Information for Clinicians,"*Ethical Human Psychology and Psychiatry* 10, no. 3 (2008): 163–78, http://findarticles.com/p/articles/mi_7530/is_200810/ai_n32305261/pg_8//

55. Rape Abuse Incest National Network, http://www.rainn.org/

56. "Frequently Asked Questions about Sexual Assault," NYU Wellness Exchange, New York University, http://www.nyu.edu/999/faqs/sexualassault.html/

57. Ibid.

58. Author interview with Howard Fradkin, November 12, 2011.

59. The National Center for Victims of Crime, "Male Rape," http://www.ncvc.org/ncvc/main.aspx?dbName=DocumentViewer&DocumentID=32361/

Selected Bibliography

Farrell, Warren. *The Myth of Male Power.* New York: Simon & Schuster, 1993.

Fillion, Kate. *Lip Service: The Truth about Women's Darker Side in Love, Sex and Friendship.* Canada: Harper Collins, 1997.

Kick, R., Editor. *Abuse Your Illusions.* New York: Disinformation Company, 2003.

Mullen, P., M. Pathé, and, R. Purcell. *Stalkers and Their Victims.* London: Cambridge University Press, 2000.

Paglia, Camille. *Vamps and Tramps.* New York: Vintage Books, 1994.

Patai, Daphne. *Heterophobia: Sexual Harassment and the Future of Feminism.* Lanham, MD: Rowman & Littlefield, 1998.

Renzetti, C.M. *Violent Betrayal: Partner Abuse in Lesbian Relationships.* Beverley Hills, CA: Sage, 1998.

Roiphe, Katie. *The Morning After: Sex, Fear and Feminism on Campus.* New York: Little Brown 1993.

Sommers, Christina Hoff. *The War Against Boys: How Misguided Feminism is Harming Our Young Men.* New York: Simon & Schuster, 2000.

Taylor, Stuart Jr., and K.C. Johnson. *Until Proven Innocent: Political Correctness and the Shameful Injustices of the Duke Lacrosse Rape Case.* New York: St. Martin's Press, 2007.

Index

About the Authors

PHILIP W. COOK is the author of *Abused Men: The Hidden Side of Domestic Violence* (Praeger/ABC-Clio, Second Edition, 2009). This volume received a number of positive reviews: "Fascinating . . . explains the many aspects of domestic violence. A wealth of material that could be helpful."—Dear Abby' Abigail Van Buren, syndicated columnist. "For a look at the often discounted issue of partner abuse against men . . . read it!"—Amy Dickinson, "Ask Amy" *Chicago Tribune* syndicated columnist. "The wife with a rolling pin is no joke, but a statistical fact . . . Cook shows at length, that the sexes have two contrasting strategies . . . By Cook's own standards, those of a journalist, this is a highly successful book."—West Coast Review of Books.

Cook is a former daily journalist who was a news director at radio stations in Portland, Oregon, and San Antonio, Texas. He also served as director of television news or assistant director of news at television stations in Reno, Nevada and Kennewick, Washington. He has received awards for his reporting from The Associated Press, The Professional Journalism Society, and the Radio Television News Directors Association. He is a graduate of the University of Oregon (1979), with a BS in Journalism.

Cook has appeared on numerous national radio and television shows such as CNN, MSNBC, Fox TV's *The Crier Report, The O'Reilly Factor* (twice), *The Montel Williams Show, The Sally Jesse Raphael Show, The Home and Family Show,* several times on the Westwood Radio Network's *Jim Bohannon Show* and CBS radio. He has been a guest on nearly 200 talk radio stations around the United States as well as being interviewed in numerous daily newspapers and the Canadian and U.S. Associated Press. His articles about domestic violence have been published in The Employee Assistance Professional "Exchange" Magazine, *The Oregonian, Women's Freedom Network Magazine, Deseret News, Eugene Register-Guard,* and many other publications. He is the co-author of articles in the distinguished academic publications *The Journal for Human Behavior in the Social Environment* and *Journal of Elder Abuse* and his articles have been published in two supplemental college textbooks, including *Domestic Violence* (2000), as well as in two anthology books published by Disinformation Press. He is the co-author of an article published in *Family Interventions in Domestic Violence,* ed. John Hamel and Tonia Nicholls (2007).

Prior to becoming an author, lecturer, and writer on domestic violence and gender issues, Cook was the executive director of the nonprofit PACE Institute For Families in Transition in Portland, Oregon. Working with two RN PhD's from Oregon Health Sciences University, a psychologist-author, and a counselor-author, the organization created the first "Children of Divorce" classes in the state. The classes taught divorcing parents how not to involve their children in disputes, how to diffuse anger, and how to support a continuing role for both parents. The demonstration classes were held for a number of years and were the subject of an hour-long prime time television special on the NBC affiliate in Portland. Eventually, the law that Mr. Cook personally wrote and helped shepherd through the legislature, allowing judges to mandate somewhat similar "Children of Divorce" classes for all divorcing parents with minor children in the state of Oregon, was signed into law (1994). The classes are now mandatory in a majority of Oregon counties.

Cook currently resides in the Portland, Oregon area. He is a writer, lecturer, and volunteers for two national organizations: Stop Abuse For Everyone, www.stopabuseforeveryone.org, and The Proposal for a White House Council on Boys and Men, www. http://whitehouse boysmen.org/blog/.

Philip W. Cook can be contacted via his website, www.abusedmen .com, or via Facebook.

TAMMY L. HODO, PhD, received her doctorate from the University of Wisconsin-Milwaukee (UWM), majoring in Urban Studies in 2009. She received her master's degree in Public Administration from Columbus State University and her bachelor's degree in Criminal Justice from Albany State University, in Georgia. Before attending UWM, she worked for the Department of Defense (Army) in Wurzburg, Germany, serving as the Administration Specialist, providing authority on manpower, personnel issues (military), Casualty Assistance and Personnel Policy. She directed personnel management programs for the Base Support Battalion (BSB); a military organization that provided community service to over 17,000 personnel who lived and worked in the Wurzburg, Germany area. While working on her PhD at UWM, Hodo worked as a project assistant for the Center for Urban Initiatives and Research (CUIR) and taught Sociology at a local community college. While working for CUIR, Hodo assisted senior researchers and staffers to develop appropriate data collection tools to evaluate pre-/post-knowledge of students enrolled in a federally funded program. Her dissertation "A Critical Analysis of an Urban Research University: Climate, Culture and Minority Faculty" was published by BiblioLabsII in 2011. Since obtaining her PhD, Hodo has worked as a Program Chair for a School of Criminal Justice while also serving as an adjunct of Sociology for the San Diego Community College System. Currently, Hodo is a dean of a technical institute and works as an adjunct in Criminal Justice at the University of the Incarnate Word in San Antonio, Texas.